Implant Excellence

Five Steps to
Grow Your Dental
Implant Practice

Implant Excellence

Five Steps to Grow Your Dental Implant Practice

Arun K. Garg, DMD

Garg Multimedia Group, Inc.
MIAMI

Garg Multimedia Group, inc.
1840 NE 153rd Street
North Miami Beach, FL 33162

©2009, 2013 Dr. Arun K. Garg, Garg Multimedia Group, Inc.
All rights reserved under all copyright conventions.

No part of this book may be reproduced, stored in a retrieval system, or transmitted by any means, electronic, mechanical, photocopying, recording, or otherwise, without written permission from Garg Multimedia Group, Inc.

ISBN: 978-0-9820953-3-1

Cover and interior design by
Robert Mott for Robert Mott & Associates
www.RobertMottDesigns.com

Printed in the United States of America.

13 14 15 16 17   10 9 8 7 6 5 4 3 2 1

Second Edition

Contents

Introduction 1

Step 1: Build a Solid Practice Foundation 7
    Chapter 1: Dare to Dream 9
    Chapter 2: Character Counts 19
    Chapter 3: The Dream Team 25
    Chapter 4: Brand You 45

Step 2: Be a Master Marketer 51
    Chapter 5: Be Your Own Marketing Expert 57
    Chapter 6: Intriguing Internal Marketing 67
    Chapter 7: Extraordinary External Marketing 79
    Chapter 8: Positive Public Relations 87
    Chapter 9: Wow Websites 97

Step 3: Make It Easy for People 107
    Chapter 10: Fantastic Phone Fundamentals 111
    Chapter 11: Creative Case Conversation: Connection 123
    Chapter 12: Creative Case Conversation: Understanding 135
    Chapter 13: Creative Case Conversation: Education 143
    Chapter 14: Creative Case Conversation: Solutions 155
    Chapter 15: Creative Case Conversation: Decision 181
    Chapter 16: Massage Money Magnificently 189

Step 4: Keep Your Promises 201
    Chapter 17: Provide Clinical Excellence 203
    Chapter 18: Stage Memorable Experiences 213

Step 5: Take Action 225
    Chapter 19: Be a Legendary Leader 227
    Chapter 20: Be Flexible in Leadership Styles 239
    Chapter 21: Capture Ideas, Set Goals 259
    Chapter 22: Seek Mastery 275

About the Author 285
Appendix A: Forms 287
Index 289

Introduction

I'M GUESSING YOU HAVE A GOOD DENTAL PRACTICE. You're earning a good living performing good dentistry on good patients. You have a good team around you, and you feel good about your life. Good for you! But maybe good isn't good enough for you right now. If that's the case, I'm committed to help you on the journey to a *great* dental practice. And increasing the amount of implants—or beginning to place implants—is a powerful tool you can use to build a great practice.

As strange as it may seem, the fact that you already have a good practice is the primary barrier to having a great one. If conditions were bad in your office right now, you would feel the sledgehammer of pain forcing you to change. But good is deceptively sneaky. It allows you to hang out in your carefully crafted comfort container, free of most discomfort but separated from greatness.

Your journey from a good to a great dental practice through implant excellence will very probably follow the storyline of a classical myth—The Hero's Journey. Countless movies and novels are based upon this meaningful legend. In it, the hero leaves his comfortable, ordinary surroundings to venture into a challenging, unfamiliar world. Part of the journey is an outer one to an actual place—a strange land (*The Wizard of Oz, Harry Potter*), the far reaches of the galaxy (*Star Wars, Star Trek*), or a new city (*Beverly Hills Cop, Rush Hour*). But the hero's story is also an inner journey of dreams, character, and spirit. The hero grows and changes, traveling from one way of life to the next—from ignorance to wisdom, from hate to love, or from weakness to strength.

Most dental practice management books are 95 to 100 percent focused on the outer journey. They tell you what you need to *do*, but not who you need to *be*. This book is about doing and being. You will learn the specific strategies you need to begin performing more implants while building a great practice, and you will discover how to be a person who attracts riches on all levels.

By the way, you should feel proud of yourself right now. It is far better to possess a good dental practice at the beginning of your journey than it is to start from a bad or an average practice, like many dentists do. Average dentists don't even read books like this one. Good is a good start. By the end of this book, you will be on your way to great.

The Conformity Coffin

I'm lucky. In my Implant Seminars presented at various locations around the country, I've met thousands of dentists. The vast majority of them are wonderful people. They mean well and want to improve themselves and their practices. But there is one thing holding them back, no matter their location or circumstances: conformity. It's far more comfortable to follow a well-worn path that thousands have followed for decades. Even though they may not have noticed it yet, these dentists are in a rut—and a rut is just a coffin with the ends kicked out.

> *A person flattened by an opponent*
> *can get up again.*
> *A person flattened by conformity*
> *stays down for good.*
>
> THOMAS WATSON

To be great is to be different; to wander away from the herd; to climb out of the conformity coffin. Luckily, the climb is simple. You just need to follow the five steps outlined in this book. But simple isn't necessarily easy. You may find that one or more of these five steps will be difficult for you to take. That's exactly why many dentists don't take them. It feels easier to stay with the herd.

I've studied the teachings of many of the great inspirational leaders of our time (Zig Ziglar, Tony Robbins, Denis Waitley, and Brian Tracy) as well as lessons imparted by past sages (Mahatma Gandhi, Albert Einstein, Albert Schweitzer, Ralph Waldo Emerson, Abraham Lincoln, Mother Teresa, and others.) As a result, much of this book is inspirational in nature. That's a good thing, since you're going to need that inspiration to keep you motivated so you can make the hard choices and complete the difficult tasks that will move you from good to great.

My Journey

After graduation from dental school and residency training, I accepted a position as assistant professor at the University of Miami Medical School. I was quickly promoted to associate professor and director of the residency training program, and soon afterwards to full professor. My rapid rise taught me two valuable lessons:

1. To be great, you have to break away from the herd. I became a full professor in less time than it usually takes.

2. Become an expert. My father was an international authority in nephrology and pharmacology. One of my mentors encouraged me to become a national authority in an area of my choosing. I decided to focus on implants, knowing my expertise in this field would lead to an emotionally and financially fulfilling career. When you become known as an implant authority in your area, your career will be enhanced, too.

I started my lecturing career speaking to local dental groups in small towns. It's a good thing the audiences were small, because I was really scared. To cover up my stage fright, I turned the lights off so no one could see me. In my early lectures, I showed 600 slides in one hour. After attending one of these, a friend of mine joked, "You could see smoke coming out of the projector!" (While my mother was always the life of the party, enjoying herself while entertaining others, I guess I didn't inherit enough of her genes.) Many people retreat when they have less-than-good experiences like that. Not me. I don't dabble in anything I do: I go all out. So I started presenting more programs at a variety of locations around the country. And, sure enough, I got better at lecturing, and pretty soon it became second nature. I could have stuck to my comfort zone and given up on public speaking, but I didn't. And it paid off.

Though I loved my 18 years at the University of Miami, enjoying intellectual stimulation in the company of other physicians, dentists, and oral surgeons, a variety of external factors led me to leave and hang out my private practice shingle. I knew the clinical aspects of bone grafting and implant dentistry inside and out, but quickly learned that my practice management skills were lacking. So I invested over $200,000 in live and remote courses to learn about practice management and personal development. I absorbed information from the best people I could find, and in typical fashion, squeezed many years of learning into just a few.

One of the best things I discovered from working with my dad was how to condense huge amounts of information into easy-to-use, bite-sized morsels. I've used this skill to create my *Implant Seminars Continuum,* to help me positively affect people's lives. My goal, which I am passionate in pursuing, is to help 1,000 general dentists per year perform better—and more—implant dentistry. If each of those dentists performs at least one implant on 100 people a year, that's 100,000 people who would benefit in the first year alone. Over time, millions of people would be positively affected. Now that gets me excited!

We're Off to See the Wizard

All heroes make an outer and inner journey, and so will you, by taking these five steps down the path to implant excellence:

Step 1: Build a Solid Practice Foundation
All structures need to have a sturdy foundation in order to stand the test of time. The same is true of your dental practice.

Step 2: Be a Master Marketer
After your foundation is in place, people will need to know about you and the implant services you provide. Otherwise, no one will benefit from your expertise.

Step 3: Make It Easy for People
Once people know about you, you must make it easy for them to accept implant dentistry by having a series of comfortable conversations with them. Now they can make the decision to benefit from your implant services.

Step 4: Keep Your Promises
You've promised patients a high level of clinical excellence and a pleasant experience. Make sure all their expectations are met.

Step 5: Take Action
You can't make the journey from good to great by yourself. You need to be an inspiring leader of a dedicated team, which means you'll need to capture the ideas that will help your team travel the path to greatness, too.

There are over 75 ideas in this book. When you find one that resonates with you, underline or highlight it. You will also generate ideas when you least expect them—at night when everyone else has gone to bed; while on a leisurely walk; or as you are peacefully sleeping. Whenever an idea pops into your mind, immediately write it down or it will return to its birthplace.

> *All the really good ideas I ever had came to me while I was milking a cow.*
> GRANT WOOD

Once you've captured these ideas, you can use them to set goals for yourself, your team, and your practice. Remember to be daring and intelligent as you complete your journey.

Conclusion

I have three sons between the ages of 11 and 17. When the best-selling book and video, *The Secret*, made it big in 2007, they told me, "Dad, this the same stuff you've been talking to us about for years. The author should have interviewed you!"

I told them, "Maybe someday, my ideas will be part of a book like *The Secret*," not knowing at the time that the first edition of this book would emerge within 18 months. In this book, you will take the journey of discovery to what I believe are the secrets of *Implant Excellence*. The journey of a thousand miles begins with a single step. Take one now and discover how to build a solid practice foundation.

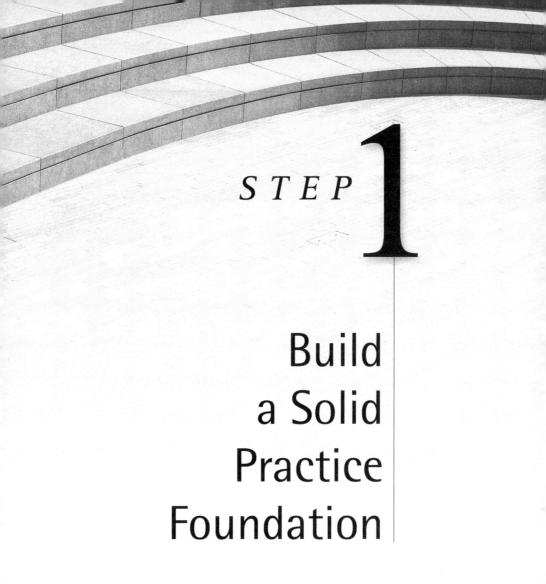

STEP 1

Build a Solid Practice Foundation

I'M SURE YOU'VE READ AND HEARD numerous stories about young singers, actors, and athletes who worked diligently to gain their fame and fortune, only to lose it by making a series of poor life choices after hitting the big time. They had talent. They had fame. Unfortunately, they didn't have a strong foundation to support their newly acquired lives.

That's why Step 1 on your journey is to build a solid practice foundation. Your foundation has four cornerstones. The first is *dreams*, which provide the inspiration for heroes to pursue their journeys. Too many dentists have given up on the dreams they had when they graduated from dental school—often, their dreams have been dashed by years of cold, hard experience. Dreams can be rekindled with new clinical skills and an enhanced outlook on life.

The second cornerstone is *character*. The development of character occurs on the inner part of the quest. Without character, behavior is haphazard and success is fleeting.

The third cornerstone is *team*. High achievers don't attain excellence by themselves. They all tap into the energy of teamwork.

The fourth cornerstone is *branding*. Like Disney, Apple, Coca-Cola, and Versace, highly successful dental practices have a habit of differentiating themselves from their competition. They create brands that attract a unique group of patients.

FOUR CORNERSTONES OF A SOLID PRACTICE FOUNDATION

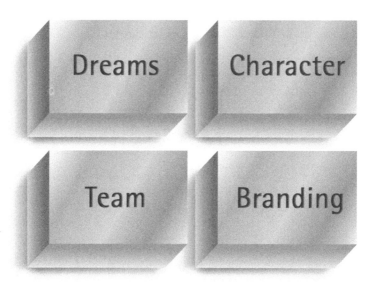

It's time to place the first cornerstone in your foundation. Turn the page, open your mind, and dare to dream.

CHAPTER 1

Dare to Dream

WALT DISNEY HAD A DREAM "To use imagination to bring happiness to millions." Dr. Martin Luther King. Jr. proclaimed, "I have a dream!"—not, "I have a strategic plan." What's your dream? What do you yearn for? What vision will propel you to rise early and stay up late to move in the direction of that dream? You've got to have a dream before you can have a dream come true. In this chapter, you will learn how to create your dream practice.

The Magic of Dreams

Dreams are magical, transforming good into great. Dreams lift people off the bench of life and propel them down new paths. The thing is, you need to be sure you're on the right path, because working harder and faster while on the wrong path will get you to a place you really don't want to go—quickly. If you're smart, it won't take you long to realize there's a better path out there, and you can look for someone to give you directions on how to get to it.

Many dentists who begin our *Implant Seminars Courses* tell me they know they must be on the wrong path. They do a little bit of dentistry on a lot of people, constantly running behind schedule as they roller skate from room to room. Their professional enjoyment level decreases as their income levels off while their overhead continues to rise. And yet, they still have mortgages to pay and families to support. What actions do you think these dentists take in their attempts to find a better path? Most sign up for more insurance plans, add more staff, and/or buy more "toys" that simply allow them to do more of the same dentistry quicker. This just makes their existing problems even worse. Busier and bigger aren't always better!

So how do you get your practice onto the right path? In our courses, we train dentists to do more high-quality, comprehensive implant dentistry on fewer patients. This is the better path, because *everyone* wins—the dentists, their teams, and their patients.

> *Our aspirations are our possibilities.*
> ROBERT BROWNING

But first, you've got to have a dream for yourself and your practice. This vision will draw you down the most ideal path like a magnet attracts iron. In addition to positioning you on the correct path:

1. **Your dream will put you on a path with other achievers and dreamers.** Ambition-deficient people sit on the bench of life and get stuck there, watching others pass by on their way to greater success. Dreamers don't have time to lollygag like that—they're going places. Once you're on your right path, you will bump into fellow dreamers on a regular basis. The achievement of your vision will be complementary with the achievement of some of your fellow travelers' dreams. Now the whole group of dreamers can work together.

    People are naturally attracted to achievers and dreamers. For example, have you ever noticed that dentists who are actively building the practice of their dreams attract the best colleagues, team members, and patients?

2. **Your dreams will bring you face to face with new opportunities and challenges.** While on your journey, you will discover new prospects that only appear to people on dream quests. You will also need to address well-timed challenges that will test your character and force you to learn new skills.

3. **Your dreams will allow you to discover catalysts that will mobilize your external resources.** You should never give up on your dream simply because you don't have the monetary and/or clinical skill resources to achieve your vision for your practice. Where there's a will, there's always a way!

Words, Images and Emotions

The mental creation of your dream practice will precede its physical creation. Life tends to give you what you think about. If you continually focus on all the negatives in your practice currently and what you *don't* want for your practice's future, life will give you more of what you don't want simply because you're concentrating on the negatives. If you form a mental creation of your dream practice on a daily basis, life will tend to move you in that direction.

The best mental creations are composed of the same three elements that director Victor Fleming used to create the 1939 movie, *The Wizard of Oz*: *words*, *images*, and *emotions*.

> **Words.** The dialogue and sound effects in *The Wizard of Oz* are hypnotically memorable. You can probably hear in your mind the Wicked Witch of the West cackling, "I'll get you, my pretty, and your little dog, too." Or Dorothy singing *Somewhere Over the Rainbow* and repeating, "There's no place like home." The words describing your dream practice and the tonality with which you say those words should be just as mesmerizing.
>
> **Images.** The images in *The Wizard of Oz* are spectacular. The dusty Kansas farm scenes were shot in black and white. The Land of Oz scenes were shot in a newly developed process called Technicolor. In your mind, do you have a vision of the twister carrying away Dorothy's house? Can you see the Cowardly Lion's face and the Scarecrow dancing? Now ask yourself, when was the last time you saw the movie? It's probably been years, maybe decades, but the images of the movie are so powerful they are burned into your memory to this day. The images you associate to your dream practice must be just as memorable and exciting.
>
> **Emotions.** Like all truly immortal movies, *The Wizard of Oz* creates a myriad of emotions: the awe at the strange and wonderful Land of Oz; the

fear of the twister and the flying monkeys; the sadness of Dorothy being left behind in Oz as the balloon sails away without her; and the joy of Dorothy returning to Kansas with the realization that "there's no place like home." People primarily do things for emotional reasons, not logical ones. This is why you must add a layer of emotion to the words and images associated with your dream practice.

Your Dream Practice Creation

> *Imagination is everything.*
> *It is the preview of life's coming attractions.*
> ALBERT EINSTEIN

Now it's time to be the director of your life and mentally create your dream practice with inspiring words, images, and emotions. You will do this in five steps.

Step One

Write your answers to the following questions in a hard-bound journal or notebook. You will use your answers at future points in this book. Notice that the questions are phrased in the *present tense*. Answer them likewise.

1. How does the exterior of your dream practice look? Picture it vividly in your mind. Walk around the office and see all the views.

2. How does the interior of your dream practice look? Picture it vividly in your mind. Walk through the office and see each room from every angle.

3. Who is working with you in the office? How many people are on the team? What are their responsibilities? Describe their temperaments, integrity, and skill sets.

4. Describe the patients who come to your practice. What services do they desire? What are their personalities like?

5. What kinds of care do you provide on a regular basis? How many implants do you place each month?

6. How many days a week are you in the practice? What are the hours? How much time do you take off for vacations and continuing education?
7. How do you look when you walk in the office's front door each morning? How does each member of your staff behave when you enter?
8. What do patients tell you about the practice?
9. What is an ideal day like in your dream practice?
10. At the end of the day, just before you fall asleep, how do you feel about your dream practice?
11. What three words most accurately describe your dream practice?

Step Two

Take all your answers and write a one-page, present-tense, dream practice description in your journal. Be sure to write what you want; not what you don't want. Let your imagination soar!

Sample Dream Practice Description

The exterior of my office building is professional—definitely a cut above. Parking is plentiful and close and shaded by flowering trees. The office interior has a definite "Wow" factor as patients walk in the door—a sleek, modern design, just like the up-to-date care we provide. Lively colors in the reception area, plenty of sunlight, comfy chairs in cheerful colors, a fully-stocked mini fridge, and unique paintings on the walls. Two private conversation areas with the latest technology to demonstrate the care we provide. Three treatment rooms are oversized and loaded with the latest equipment. My private office is tastefully decorated—an oasis for me, with plants, artwork, an ergonomic chair, and the latest laptop computer on my mahogany desk. A large area for our team to get together, with a round table we can all sit around as equal participants.

There are four other members on the team—a front desk person, two clinical nurses/assistants, and a hygienist, all people I enjoy being with. We have a blast and include our patients in the fun. We see an average of six hygiene, four new, and two surgical patients a day. Our patients desire the best care available and are willing to pay for it. They are pleasant to care for. Difficult people are referred to other offices. We provide only the most advanced implant and related hard and soft tissue grafting procedures. We place an average of 80 implants a month on an average of 10 patients a month.

Most weeks we are in the office on Tuesday and Thursday from 9:00 am to 4:30 pm with an hour for lunch. On Wednesday, our office hours are 8:30 am to 8:30 pm with an hour for lunch. Occasionally we do a big case on Monday, Friday or Saturday. We are in the office 45 weeks a year. We take off seven weeks each year for vacations and continuing education.

I walk in the office door each day with a big smile on my face. I love coming here. The patients are really our friends. They tell us ours is the best dental office they have ever been to and enthusiastically refer their family and friends.

Our ideal day is relaxed yet challenging. We are almost always running on or ahead of schedule. We have time to do the best implant dentistry possible. The day is a wonderful experience for everyone involved. At the end of the day, the entire team leaves together.

When I fall asleep at night, I'm grateful for having such a rewarding practice. Three words that describe my practice are modern, fun, and fulfilling.

Step Three

Read your dream practice description out loud a few times to fix it in your mind. Don't memorize it. Just read the description with emotion.

Step Four

Silently read your dream practice description once, early in the day. Then close your eyes and picture all the images associated with the words from beginning to end. Make the images big, bright, and colorful—just like the Land of Oz. Be sure to add movement and a soundtrack to the images. In addition to the images, hear, taste, smell and touch everything around you. Use all five of your senses to create a memorable experience. Add more and more specific details if you want—the exact color of the walls, floors, chairs, etc.

> *Champions aren't made in the gyms.*
> *Champions are made from something*
> *they have deeper inside them—*
> *a desire, a dream, a vision.*
> *They have last-minute stamina.*
> *They have to be a little faster.*
> *They have to have the skill and the will.*
> *But the will must be stronger than the skill.*
>
> MUHAMMAD ALI

Step Five

In the *Wizard of Oz*, the Munchkins gave Dorothy very simple yet profound advice: "Follow the Yellow Brick Road. Follow the Yellow Brick Road. Follow, follow, follow, follow, follow the Yellow Brick Road." They knew that it was best for Dorothy not to focus on her goal of reaching the Emerald City (a vision to be reached in the future), but to focus on one step at a time down the Yellow Brick Road (a series of actions in the present).

As you go through your day, do the same. Forget about your dream practice. That's right. Just forget about it and live each moment of the day in the present. Act like Dorothy and consider your life as a series of simple, single steps—"now" moments—strung together. What you think and do each moment casts a spell (for better or worse) over the moments that follow. By having a dream and keeping your attention in the here and now, everything you desire in life will spontaneously flow to you instead of you grasping for it. *Having* anything in life is simply a matter of focusing your attention on *being* (the subject of the next chapter), *doing,* and *giving.* Relax and let life automatically create your desire.

> *Success is like a butterfly.*
> *The more you chase it,*
> *The more it eludes you.*
> *But if you turn your attention to other things,*
> *It comes softly and sits on your shoulder.*
> ANONYMOUS

Don't Be Dangerous: Be Smart

We've all heard the stories of dentists proceeding at breakneck speed down the wrong path—dentists who, in their zeal to create high-end cosmetic practices, severely damage their traditional family practices. These dentists are good people who believe in their dreams. They're excited about creating the kind of practice that's glowingly described in the magazines. They work hard and invest huge sums of money in equipment and training. They're excited, but they're on the wrong path because they don't know what they're doing. People who are excited but don't know what they're doing are dangerous for their practice!

Don't be dangerous. Be smart instead, by taking great care of your traditional practice as you do more and more implant cases. At first, the patients desiring implants are going to be established patients from your traditional family practice. If you alienate your established patients, who are you going to discuss implants with? As you intelligently and gradually create a growing group of implant patients in your community, your reputation as an expert will grow. Then you will begin to attract patients who want that type of dentistry from outside your traditional practice. Eventually, as you perform an increasing number of implants, you can morph your traditional family or general practice into a high-end implant practice. When you allow this morphing to naturally occur, there's no need to force the issue. You also can stop the morphing process at any point in time—not all dentists want high-end implant practices. You can create a dream practice that is perfect for you, with the right blend of traditional and implant cases to suit your needs.

Conclusion

By daring to dream, you have put the first cornerstone of your solid practice foundation in place. By themselves, however, dreams are not enough. You must have the character needed to proceed with passion and purpose down the right path to your dream. Follow your yellow brick road right now and see why your character counts.

CHAPTER 2
Character Counts

I OCCASIONALLY MEET DENTISTS who lament, "I can never find good people to work for me. I've looked everywhere; and there are no qualified people out there. And patients these days don't want to spend any money on comprehensive dentistry. They just want to patch things up and have the very minimum done."

I don't say this, but I'm thinking, "Perhaps it's not them. Maybe it's you!" I know there are times when the "people part" of dentistry is a challenge, but if it's *always* that way, the dentists should think twice about blaming their external circumstances. They should check their internal character and realize that while their words *speak* to people, their character *shouts* at them.

> *Everyone thinks of changing the world,*
> *but no one thinks of changing himself.*
> LEO TOLSTOY

Focus on the Internal First

We frequently allow our character to block us from all the emotional and financial riches the world has to offer. For example, when most dentists think about hiring team members and attracting patients, they focus on *external* factors such as placing good ads in the right places and using the best hiring procedures. While these external factors are important, they pale in comparison to *internal* factors like the dentist's own character.

> *Character is what you have left*
> *when you've lost everything you can lose.*
> EVAN ESAR

People want to work with dentists who are honest, caring, enthusiastic, and fair. They want to work with leaders, not serve under dictators. They want to be players on a team rather than workers on a staff. They want to enjoy helping their employers instead of just tolerating them. Likewise, patients seek to visit dental offices where the dentists are caring, not aloof; personable, not distant; and friendly, not abrupt. For high-end dental care, patients need to know you are the right *person* before they want to hear about the right dentistry. They look to the inner first and the outer later.

The Character–Action Connection

The firefighters and police officers who rushed into the burning World Trade Center on September 11, 2001 did so because that's just who they are. When their captains led them on rescue missions into the towering infernos, even though it was obviously dangerous, the rescuers didn't have to think long and hard about their behavior. They just did it. Their character traits—bravery and self-sacrifice—automatically created their actions.

> *Character is doing what's right*
> *when nobody's looking.*
> J.C. WATTS

The connection between character and action is automatic. Honest people just tell the truth—there's no conscious thought involved. Caring people spontaneously show thoughtfulness with their words and deeds. Disciplined people have a servo-mechanism that produces goal-oriented behavior day in and day out.

The Character Question

As you can see, the character traits you possess are vitally important to your success. So answer the question, "What are the five most important character traits I need in order to create and maintain my dream practice?" (For the best answer, first review the dream practice description you created in the last chapter.) As an example, to create and maintain your dream practice you believe you will need to be caring, ethical, and disciplined, curious and outgoing. Then, in your journal or notebook, write each of the character traits at the top of a different page. Leave the rest of each page blank for now.

> *Good character is more to be praised*
> *than outstanding talent.*
> *Most talents are, to some extent, a gift.*
> *Good character, by contrast, is not given to us.*
> *We have to build it piece by piece,*
> *by thought, courage and determination.*
>
> JOHN LUTHER

Character Trait Tools

You have three tools with which to build your character, whether you're starting over or just improving yourself: *focus, action,* and *surroundings.*

> **Focus.** Have you ever watched professional golfers play in a tournament on TV? As they walk around the golf course, they aren't focusing on the crowds of spectators, or the scenic views, or the cameras. They simply focus on the key aspects of their environment that give them the information needed to hit the next shot well. Your $64,000 question is, "What key aspects should I focus on to create my dream practice?" Determine which parts of your world will enjoyably reinforce the character traits you've identified. Then focus on these parts of your world.

> *What we notice becomes our world.*
> PATRICIA RYAN MADSON

Action. Your second character creation tool is action. In a reciprocal fashion, character produces behavior and behavior builds character. To create a specific character trait, act like a person who already has that trait. One of the best ways to illustrate this point: put a smile on your face the next time you're in bad mood. No matter how fake that smile is, you'll find it's difficult to maintain a grumpy feeling for very long.

> *We are what we pretend to be.*
> *So we must be careful what we pretend to be.*
> KURT VONNEGUT

Surroundings. The people and places that make up your environment shape your character. As such, you need to carefully choose the people with whom you associate and the settings you frequent. If you belong to a group with dentists who constantly complain about how bad their practices are but who aren't taking actions that could improve them, you need to find a new group. If the people on your office team aren't actively supporting the creation of your dream practice, you must make constructive changes to your staff. If the design and décor of your office doesn't exemplify the quality of dentistry your dream practice will provide, it's vital that you make the necessary improvements now.

> *Choose the environment that will best develop*
> *you toward your objective.*
> *Analyze your life in terms of its environment.*
> *Are the things around you helping you toward success;*
> *or are they holding you back?*
> W. CLEMENT STONE

Building Each Character Trait

Now that you've selected the five most important character traits required to create and maintain your dream practice and written each one at the top of a different page in your journal or notebook, you're ready for the next step. Under each character trait, write how you will use focus, action, and surroundings to build that trait. Here are three examples:

Caring

I'm a caring dentist who focuses on the patient's best interests at all times. I make the effort to discover people's unique fears and desires. I spend extra time talking with them about non-dental topics. I smile and respectfully touch patients as I would a friend. I take communication and personal development courses and implement what I learn. I surround myself with a team of caring people who reinforce the impressions that I've given patients. I have a room in the office where my team and I can talk with our patients privately.

Ethical

I'm an ethical dentist who focuses on doing the right things. Keeping in mind their financial circumstances, I always do what is best for my patients. I educate my patients so they can appreciate the best that dentistry has to offer. I never lie or shade the truth. I do what I say I will do. When appropriate, I offer a variety of treatment options, explain the advantages and disadvantages of each option, and make my recommendation. I surround myself with highly ethical people and provide career adjustments to those who aren't.

Disciplined

I'm a disciplined dentist who focuses on the path leading to my dream practice. I learn whatever clinical, practice management, communication, and leadership tools I will need. I do whatever it takes to build my dream practice. I create a weekly schedule which I follow closely. I surround myself with disciplined people.

There is no right or wrong when it comes to your dream practice, the character traits on your list, and the tools you use to achieve them. Even traits like "ruthless" and "relentless" can be positive if you apply them correctly, as in "the ruthless or relentless pursuit of continuing education and skill improvement." Make sure your creation is not a carbon copy of someone else's dream practice. You're a unique individual. Your dream practice and character should be unique, too.

> *Most people are other people.*
> *Their thoughts are someone else's opinions,*
> *their lives a mimicry, their passions a quotation.*
>
> OSCAR WILDE

Conclusion

Mahatma Gandhi said, "You must be the change you wish to see in people." Truer words were never spoken. If you want your team to change for the better, you must demonstrate the change first. If you want your patients to change their opinions of implant dentistry, you must change first.

In this chapter, you learned how to change a vital part of your being—your character. In the next chapter, you will discover how to create a group of people who will work together to help each other achieve their collective dreams. Your dream team is poised to take the field, so read on to learn how to coach them.

CHAPTER 3

The Dream Team

DID YOU SEE the 2013 Academy Award winning movie, *Argo*? It was a terrific flick because an inspiring story was magnificently told by a team of extremely talented people. The producers, George Clooney, Ben Affleck and Grant Heslov, put together the team including screenplay writer, Chris Terrio, and actors Alan Arkin and John Goodman. Ben directed and starred in the feature. In addition, there were hundreds of other highly skilled and passionate people who had key parts in the movie-making. Argo cost $44M to make. The worldwide box office was $232M!

Do you have an equally effective dream team—a "Team You"? I hope so, because you will need a lot of assistance on the journey to your dream practice. It's also important to realize that Team You isn't just your office team. It's also your family, sales reps, colleagues, mentors, teachers, friends, and heroes. Like the different keys on a piano, they are all needed to create virtuoso dental implant excellence.

Hire for Attitude and Train for Skill

Every person views the world with varying degrees of positive and negative attitudes. Some people view the world through negative attitudes. As a result, they see the negative in the world, do negative things, and achieve negative results... which, of course, reinforces their negative attitudes. Avoid these people like the plague. You may believe in your ability to change their attitudes, but 98 percent of the time you will be wrong—and your own attitude may be pulled into the dumpster as well.

Other people view the world through their positive attitudes. These are the folks you want as members of your office team. Unfortunately, attitude is not given due respect when employers are seeking and selecting employees. While skills can be learned—especially by enthusiastic, optimistic people—attitudes are more pervasive qualities that typically are fixed by the time adulthood rolls around.

Combining Attitude and Skill

Based on the variables of (1) attitude and (2) skill, four possible groups are created.

1. **Positive Attitude/High Skill.** These gems make the greatest contribution to your practice. Therefore, hiring and retaining them is your first priority. These individuals are rare, in demand, and command the best pay. But pay is not their greatest reward: they must also feel appreciated and remain professionally stimulated. Make sure you search for them during your new team selection process.

2. **Positive Attitude/Low Skill.** These highly motivated individuals are the next best bet for your practice. Consider these individuals as diamonds in the rough. They have great potential to grow into the skill level that the job demands—all you need to do is educate them.

3. **Negative Attitude/High Skill.** These are the people who drain your energy and keep you awake at night. They may have great skill, but they are overly critical of other team members whom they don't feel are living up to their high standards. (Make sure you are not in this group yourself!)

4. **Negative Attitude/Low Skill.** If one of these individuals is currently on or eventually surfaces on your team, sever the relationship as soon as possible.

Wondering how to find, select, and keep people with the best attitudes as part of your office team? You're in the right place—read on.

Find People with Great Attitudes

It's a basic truth: you attract what you deserve in life. If you're a lousy dentist with a lousy practice, you're going to attract lousy team members. If you're an average dentist with an average practice, you're going to attract average team members. If you're an outstanding dentist with an outstanding practice, you're going to attract outstanding team members. This is great news! If your success was primarily due to external factors, there wouldn't be much you could do to improve the situation. But once you've improved your own attitude and developed the positive character traits you identified in the last chapter, you'll begin attracting better candidates.

Here are four ways to find people with great attitudes:

1. Start by reviewing your patient list to see if there are any contenders. Note the patients that your team loves to see walk in the door.

2. Interview friends of team members with great attitudes. Like birds of a feather, people with positive attitudes tend to flock together.

3. Always be on the lookout. Whenever you run into a particularly friendly person in any service situation—a restaurant, retail store, etc.—invite them to the office for an interview.

4. Don't run the same uninspiring classified ads every other dentist in town is using. Be clear up front that you're looking for positive people to be part of a team that values great attitudes and has fun at work.

Here are some actual, positive-attitude-attracting ads I've seen. You may find them a little unusual—which is necessary if you want to attract unusual people.

Hygienist

Very progressive dental office seeking enthusiastic, positive, ambitious hygienist with team-player mentality, exceptional verbal skills, & dynamic personality. Full-time, excellent hours, 4 days/week (M-Th 8am-5 pm), great pay with built-in bonus system. Please call xxx-xxx-xxxx.

Front Office

We are looking for a positive person for the front office of our dental practice. We are selective on who we treat, so we are selective on who we hire. We need someone that dresses professionally as you will be greeting all of our patients as they enter. We need someone with enough life experience to know that they are fortunate to be on our team and can relay this good fortune to all that enter. We need someone energetic and passionate about what they do, all with a smile.

We are a small team, with only one person up front (this position), which means you need experience in this capacity. We are a low volume, low stress team that deals with more elective procedures. We are not anti-insurance, but we don't run an insurance mill, so stress is controlled. We are not PPO providers. We accept assignment of benefits, but don't routinely submit for pre-determinations (insurance is a benefit, not a focus).

Our fees are paid in advance, so we are looking for someone that values dentistry enough to ask for large sums in advance of treatment. Our fees are in the 95th percentile, so you will hear comments about us being expensive. We are worth it, and you must agree.

We work 160 days per year, 30-35 hours per week. We take two-hour lunches on Mondays and Tuesdays, but skip lunch Wednesday and Thursday so we can leave early and beat the traffic. We run on time. If you are chronically 3 minutes late, don't apply.

This is not an entry-level position, but it is not managerial either. The level of customer service that we are looking for is experienced at Nordstrom or Neiman Marcus. We need the phones answered, the schedule filled and money collected. Call xxx-xxxx to schedule a visit.

GENERAL AD #1

Are you an experienced (position) who loves being optimistic, enjoys problem solving and is proactive? Do you dream of working for a dentist who encourages you to have input, feedback, AND appreciates you for what you do? If you are optimistic, energetic, proactive, and a problem solver, please fax your resume to xxx-xxx-xxxx.

GENERAL AD #2

Are you the (position) of our dreams? We are looking for the best (position) to take care of the greatest patients and work with the most outstanding dental team! If you want to contribute your skills, knowledge, talent, and personality to our organization, please let us know by faxing your resume to xxx-xxx-xxxx.

GENERAL AD #3

Are you the SUPERSTAR of our dreams?

We are looking for a dynamic (position) to take care of the greatest patients in the world, while working with the most outstanding dental team. Our successful (city) office specializes in general, cosmetic, and implant dentistry. If you want to be richly rewarded for your skills, knowledge, talent and personality, please fax your resume to (xxx) xxx-xxxx.

Select People with Great Attitudes

Now that you've found a few people who appear to have great attitudes, it's time to select the candidate possessing the best combination of positive attitude and high skill. Your selection process should go far beyond finding someone who looks good, sounds good, and can work the necessary hours. Bringing the wrong person into your practice can be a bad experience for everyone involved. The person, your team, and you won't be happy, and it will cause your patients to wonder, "Why does the doc have a different group of people working here every time I come in to have my teeth cleaned?"

To maximize your chances of selecting the right person, use the following nine-step process.

1. Before inviting candidates into your office for a personal interview, be sure someone in your office talks with them on the phone. If they don't sound good over the phone, I can almost guarantee they won't be good in person.

2. One trusted office team member (not you) should sit down with each applicant in a private area and have a conversation. In addition to reviewing their resumes and asking the usual questions about skill and experience, inquire about their lives. What do they enjoy doing in their spare time? What is their favorite television program? What was the last book they read? What people do they most admire? What's most important to them in life? What's most important to them in a job/occupation? What's one valuable thing they've learned in the past week? Pay attention to *what* they're saying and *how* they say it. Do they have an infectious smile and seem eager to learn? Are they excited about life and the opportunity to work in your office? Is this someone who would be a joy to work with for seven, eight, or ten hours a day?

3. Ask them, "What were the people like in the last office you worked in?" Most of the time, they will think the same things about your team. Listen very carefully to their answers.

4. Evaluate their humor index with these questions: "How have you recently used humor in a work environment? Have you ever used humor to diffuse a difficult situation? What's one of your favorite jokes or funny stories?"

5. Quickly, assess gut feeling about their attitudes. On a low-to-high scale of 1 to 10, where do they stand? Only consider those who are at 8, 9, or 10.

6. Have each person come back to the office to briefly meet with you and then go to lunch with the team (minus you).

7. As a team, evaluate the personality assessment and everyone's impressions. In most cases, the dental team does a better job of picking excellent new team members than the doctor.

8. Complete reference and background checks on your top candidate. (You can do these checks yourself, or contact me for recommendations.)

9. Have the top candidate back for a one-week, paid, working interview. At the end of the week make the decision to offer the person a permanent position—or not.

Keep People with Great Attitudes

Now that you've selected people with great attitudes, you need to keep them. Here are my top eight ways to hold on to highly valued employees.

1. **Model the attitude you want to see in your team.** You can't expect them to have great attitudes if you don't. Many dental teams' attitudes are the mirror image of their doctor's attitude. If you don't like what you see in your team, look in the mirror for a probable cause.

2. **Surround your team with competent people who have great attitudes.** People with great attitudes prefer being around others with great attitudes. If you have a person on your team with a bad attitude, have a talk or two with the person. If they don't change, give them a career adjustment. Do you have someone on your team whose personality is "iffy?" If the answer is, "Yes," ask yourself this question, "Knowing what I now know about this person, would I hire them again?" If your answer to that question is, "No," give them the opportunity to find employment elsewhere.

3. **Create a practice vision that your team will buy into.** In the first chapter, you created a dream practice with sounds, images, and emotions. It's vital that you communicate this dream to your team. People with great attitudes want to know your vision of your practice, what role they play and how they too will benefit from the achievement of

your dream.

4. **Expect the best from your team.** In an experiment, several teachers were each given a class of students and told, "Your students are highly intelligent. They have very high IQs and are capable of achieving outstanding results in school." The second group of teachers were each given classes of students and told, "Your students have average IQs and scholastic ability. We expect only average results from them." As expected, the "highly intelligent" students did far better than the average students. The amazing thing was that all the classes of students were average—there were no "highly intelligent" students. The only difference was what the teachers expected from their students. A similar result will occur in your office when you expect the best from your team.

A great way to communicate that you expect the best from your team is to add the phrase "and whatever it takes to give outstanding service to all our patients" to the end of everyone's job descriptions. Stress the "whatever it takes" concept to your team. Make it a big deal. Talk about it over and over.

> *Treat people as though*
> *they were what they ought to be*
> *and you help them become*
> *what they are capable of being.*
>
> GOETHE

5. **Recognize, reward, and praise your team.** Some dentists take "The Firings Will Continue Until Moral Improves" approach to motivating their teams. The majority of dentists care about the people they work with, but they are often too busy, too stressed, or don't have enough good ideas to make their staff feel appreciated on a regular basis. Employers often don't realize how important the warm, fuzzy things are to their teams. In a series of studies, it was discovered that the things managers perceived as being most important to employees were vastly different to what the employees reported as being desirable.

Below is a chart of 10 factors people could desire in a job and how managers and employees ranked each of the 10.

Factor	Managers	Employees
Good wages	1	5
Job security	2	4
Promotion/growth opportunities	3	7
Good working conditions	4	9
Interesting work	5	6
Personal loyalty to employees	6	8
Tactful disciplining	7	10
Full appreciation of work done	8	1
Sympathetic to personal problems	9	3
Feeling "in" on things	10	2

As you can see from the rankings above, the managers' bottom three rankings were the employees' top three rankings. It's interesting to note that all three factors fall into the "warm, fuzzy" category and have nothing to do with money.

So how often are employees receiving the factor they ranked topmost—full appreciation of work done? Take a look at these statistics taken from a study of 1,500 corporate employees done by Dr. Gerald Graham :

- 58 percent said they seldom, if ever, received personal thanks from their manager
- 76 percent said they seldom, if ever, received written thanks from their manager
- 81 percent said they seldom, if ever, received public praise in the workplace
- 92 percent said they seldom, if ever, participated in morale-building meetings

Here are two ways to reward your dental team. For others, please contact me for book recommendations.

Compliment People with this Four-Step Process

1. Compliment people as soon as possible after the behavior.
2. Begin the compliment with the person's name.
3. Compliment a specific action. It's important the people being complimented link the praise to a specific action taken. Now they know exactly what to do again.
4. Explain why the action was important to you. This step adds extra impact to the compliment.

Here's an example of an effective compliment to a clinical assistant: "Sam, you did a wonderful job just now of helping calm Larry down. That's just the kind of service we like to give here in the office."

Write Thank-You Notes to Your Team

In addition to thanking your team with words, I hope you give them written thank-you notes too. The notes can be as simple as a sticky note with the words "Thanks for being such a wonderful member of our team" placed in an area where the person will see it first thing in the morning. Or the notes can be written on cards purchased at stationery or office supply stores. Here's a template you can follow:

> Charlotte:
>
> I really enjoy having you on our team. I'd like to thank you for *(pick one of the following)*:
> - believing in my dream practice and me. You are an important part of making the dream come true.
> - your dedication. You've been with us for three years now, and I feel like you're part of the family.
> - your commitment to our patients. I have so much confidence in you and your abilities.
> - your honesty and commitment to open and supportive communication. I truly value your integrity.
>
> I've really enjoyed working with you the past three years, and I look forward to many more. Thanks for being on the team!
>
> *Your Signature*

Good thoughts not delivered mean squat.

KEN BLANCHARD

6. **Provide your team with extensive training.** People with great attitudes constantly want to grow professionally and personally. Help them develop by regularly providing books, audios, and videos on clinical, service, and personal development topics. Hold team meetings where the team members or you provide professional and personal development information. Take your team with you when attending meetings and conferences.

7. **Give your team enhanced responsibilities.** People with great attitudes thrive on having enhanced responsibilities. In order for this to occur, your staff must first have been given comprehensive training to effectively handle the enhanced responsibilities given them. Second, you must step back and give them the freedom to do

their jobs. Until you embrace this two-step process, you won't effectively move toward the creation of your dream practice.

8. **Make office enjoyment a priority.** Think about all the numbers you track, compile, and analyze at the end of each month. Are your measurements a long list of logical items such as number of new patients, gross production, net income, and accounts receivable? While these numbers are important, I believe they omit one vital aspect of your practice that rarely is measured and prioritized: the enjoyment level of the entire team.

   Here's what I recommend you do. Once a month, at one of your regular meetings, have everyone rate their experience in the office the past 30 days on a scale of -10 to +10.

   - **-10 represents,** "I absolutely hate my time in the office!"
   - **0 represents,** "My time in the office is okay."
   - **+10 represents,** "I absolutely love my time in the office!"

   Add all the numbers and divide by the number of team members to get an average score. Then have the team members answer these questions:

   a. **What happened last month that positively affected our enjoyment level?** As an example, "We did a lot of implant cases last month. The patient visits were longer, and we weren't so rushed."

   b. **How can we expand upon this to increase our enjoyment level?** As an example, "Let's improve our plan to present implant dentistry to new and recare patients."

   c. **What happened last month that negatively affected our enjoyment level?** As an example, "We squeezed in our emergency patients at the end of day about 30 percent of the time. As a result, we were late leaving the office on many occasions."

   d. **How can we prevent or lessen this in the future to increase our enjoyment level?** As an example, "Let's set aside an extra 15 minutes at the end of the day for emergencies."

Now, take action on your answers. Assign one person to be in charge of each action item and set a completion date for each action item. That's true teamwork that allows each staff member to feel part of a team, not part of a machine.

Develop Strengths and Manage Weaknessess

We're all born with a unique set of talents and weaknesses. Talents are the activities where we naturally shine, and weaknesses are the areas where we have challenges. To be an effective leader, you must soar with your strengths and manage your weaknesses... and help your team do the same.

Talent must be cultivated. It needs to be developed. If not, people go through their lives with latent potential, but don't use their talents as fully as they should. When that happens, everyone loses.

> *As tools become rusty, so does the mind;*
> *a garden uncared for soon becomes smothered*
> *in weeds; a talent neglected withers and dies.*
> ETHEL PAGE

Three Myths about Talents and Weaknesses

In their book, *Soar With Your Strengths,* Donald Clifton and Paula Nelson discuss the myths associated with talents and weaknesses. Here, in modified form, are three of them.

Myth #1 - Fixing weaknesses creates excellence

It's a big mistake to focus all attention on fixing weaknesses. This will improve the performance of a person or company, but it will not create greatness. For example, a weakness of many dentists is that we aren't business oriented. They may be creative and have high levels of manual dexterity, but they lack the business orientation talent.

If they dramatically improved their business skills, would they be excellent dentists? No. At best they would be better dentists. And if the dentists focused almost all of their attention on business skills and neglected the clinical, leadership and communication skills, they might even decrease their over-all effectiveness.

> *If a man does not keep pace with his companions, perhaps he hears a different drummer.*
>
> HENRY DAVID THOREAU

Myth #2: Talents don't require attention: They take care of themselves

Myth #2 is a corollary to #1. Traditional thinking says that, if you want to excel, don't waste your time on improving your talents. Instead, put your time into improving your weak areas. Clifton and Nelson describe a study where over 1,000 college students were tested and placed into one of two groups—slow readers or fast readers. Both groups then took the same speed-reading training course. The slow readers went from an average of 90 words per minute to 150 words per minute after the training—a respectable 67% increase. To the astonishment of the researchers, the fast readers went from an average of 350 words per minute before the course to more than 2,900 words per minute afterwards—a 728% increase! The moral: Talents do require attention to reach their maximum potential.

Myth #3: Everyone can do anything they set their minds to

Myth #3 sounds good when you first hear it. But belief in this myth can lead to discouragement and disillusionment. Myth #3 creates the notion that you can accomplish anything if you just work hard enough at it. This myth is supported by several popular sayings. Here they are, followed by what I believe is a more accurate statement.

- *"If they can do it, so can you."* This should be, **"If they can do it, those with the same natural talents in similar situations can, too."**
- *"If at first you don't succeed, try, try again."* This should be, **"If at first you don't succeed, make sure you have the natural talents to succeed."**

- *"If you conceive it and believe it, then you will achieve it."* This should be, **"If you conceive it and believe it, you may achieve it—if it employs your talents and the time is right."**

Discovering Talents

So, how do you discover talents in your team, your children and yourself? Here are four ways.

1. Pay attention to deeply held desires

The word *desire* comes from the Latin word *desiderare,* which means "from the stars." As a leader, what stars do your team members want to touch? I'm guessing one of their natural talents is wrapped up in that desire. Listen for the expression of their desires. Then put them in situations where they can best express their talents.

You also must watch out for dead-end desires—those desires that take you in directions away from the use of your natural talents. When they first enter the profession, some dentists' dead-end desires are money and prestige. They don't consider the fact that being a dentist doesn't play into their natural talents. They may make the money and have the prestige, but they're miserable in the process.

Finally, be aware of what others think you should do with your life. They may not be considering your talents. Too many people are living someone else's visions for their lives instead of considering what their natural talents and desires lead them to. Make sure the life you live is the one you want.

> *My role is about unleashing what people*
> *already have inside them*
> *that is maybe suppressed in most work environments.*
>
> **TONY HSIEH**
> FOUNDER OF ZAPPOS

2. Be alert for fulfillment

What activities bring you the most fulfillment? What parts of your day seem to fly by and don't feel like work at all? I'll bet a talent is working behind the scenes.

As a leader, notice the times when your team members are fulfilled. Then give them the opportunity to spend more time doing those activities. This will allow them to soar with their strengths. Everybody—the person, the patient, your practice, and you—will benefit.

3. Notice rapid learning

As you learned earlier, the students who were naturally good at reading improved the most when given training. What activities did you learn quickly in your life? A talent was probably in play. At work, what activities do team members pick up quickly? Those activities play to their talents. Have them do more in that area.

> *To do easily what is difficult for others is the mark of talent.*
>
> HENRI-FRÉDÉRIC AMIEL

4. Identify snapshots of excellence

Out of the blue, have you ever done something in a fabulous fashion? Has a person in your practice done the same? That snapshot of excellence may be revealing a hidden talent. Capitalize on your discovery. When it comes to talents, the bottom line is this: Discover what you do best, and then do more of it. In your practice, discover what the people you lead and manage do best, and then allow them to do more of it.

Discovering Weaknesses

Don't get me wrong: when it comes to weaknesses, I'm not saying that you should never work on them. I am saying that there will come a point in time when the rewards you receive from working on weaknesses won't be worth the effort. If you're a superb clinical dentist, but you're not great at financials, you can work hard to familiarize yourself with basic accounting principles. But there will come a point when learning the details of financial spreadsheets probably won't be the best use of your time. The same goes with the people you lead at work.

Weaknesses are painfully easy to detect: Simply review the activities you routinely do and answer these three questions:

1. Is learning this particular activity difficult and slow?
2. Do you dislike doing the activity?
3. Do you feel burned out performing the activity?

If the answer to one or more of the questions is "yes", the activity is a weakness for you. Now you need to learn how to manage it.

Managing Weaknesses

Your goal is not to ignore your weaknesses. Your goal is to manage weaknesses so your strengths can be unleashed and become so powerful, they make the weaknesses irrelevant. Here are four ways to manage a weakness.

1. **Let it go.** This is easier said than done. Sometimes we get stuck in patterns that don't support us. Try letting a weakness go for a month. Then decide if it was a good choice.

2. **Let someone else do it.** When it comes to home repairs and home improvements, I let someone else do it. I don't enjoy doing the repairs and improvements, and I'm not good at it. What activities in your personal and professional lives fall into the same category? How will you give these activities to someone else?

3. **Form partnerships.** The best relationships are those where the strengths of the partners complement each other. In show business, Cher had singing talent, and Sonny had business talent. Neither of them would probably have made it on their own in the beginning. What partnerships will improve your personal life and business?

4. **Create support systems.** What support systems do you need in your personal life and profession? The support could come from your family, your team, your friends, or coaches and consultants.

When it comes to weaknesses, the bottom line is this: Discover what you don't do well and stop doing it or do less of it. In dentistry, discover what the people you lead don't do well and allow them to do the same.

Maybe you can teach a turkey to climb a tree,
but you're probably better off
hiring a squirrel in the first place.

KATHY MURPHY

Realize That Everybody Has Unique Talents

The realization that all members of your business team have natural talents that can be developed with training and experience is a huge advantage for you. If every day you walked past your compressor, and it was running at sixty percent efficiency, what would you do to enhance its performance? Almost anything, right? Many of the people you walk past in your practice each day are like that machine. Their talents aren't being utilized to maximum effectiveness. And it's negatively affecting the bottom line of your practice far more than a broken piece of machinery.

There are two ways of being creative.
One can sing and dance.
Or one can create an environment
in which singers and dancers flourish.

WARREN BENNIS

A recent study showed that only 16% of employees said they used more than half of their talents at work. Imagine what your office would be like if everyone's talents were tapped at a high level. They would experience the joy and juice of doing their *best* work, not just *good* work. And your practice would reap the rewards. Make talent identification and development an integral part of doing business. Promote it. Reward it. Then, sit back and watch an enthusiastic and talented group of people achieve extraordinary results.

Personality Assessments

Like talents, an adult personality is rather rigid. Personality assessments such as the Myers-Briggs are excellent methods to evaluate your team's and your personality types. Be sure you use any personality assessment as an additional tool to gain *insight* into personality. Contact me if you need guidance on where to find these.

Conclusion

I believe the formation of a dream team is one of the most important actions you can take as a business owner. Clooney, Affleck and Heslov know full well the value of team. And their *Argo* bet paid off handsomely for them.

Branding, the subject of the next chapter, is rarely discussed in dentistry today. To many dentists, the topic of branding seems unprofessional and too commercial. By reading Chapter 4, I believe you will find branding to be very professional and highly personal. Have I piqued your interest? I hope so. Flip the page and discover the power of Brand You.

CHAPTER 4

Brand You

There are four cornerstones to implant excellence. In Chapter 1, you placed the first cornerstone—dreams. You created the practice of your dreams in words, images, and emotions. In Chapter 2, you placed the second cornerstone—character. You identified the five character traits needed to move toward your dream practice and created a plan to build each trait with focus, action, and surroundings. In Chapter 3, you placed the third cornerstone—team. You discovered how to find, select, and keep skillful people with great attitudes to be members of your implant excellence team.

In this chapter, you will place the fourth and final cornerstone—branding.

The Power of Branding

Apple is the #1 brand in the world with a brand value of $87 billion! The average Apple Store sells $6,000 per square foot each year. This is double of its nearest competitor—Tiffany. There are 3,000 square feet in an Apple Store. So each location sells $18 million per year!

There are many definitions of a brand. My favorite is: **a brand consists of the words, images, and emotions in the mind of the public that are attached to an entity such as a business, location, or person.** What words, images, and emotions pop into your mind when you hear the following?

- A place where unusual and high-quality coffee drinks are prepared your way by caring people in a comfortable atmosphere
- A kingdom of dreams where imagination and fantasy go hand in hand, spreading smiles and laughter to children of all ages
- A city where anything goes, a place where you can do the crazy things you would never do at home—and nobody will hear about it
- A sports shoe, apparel, and equipment company that allows you to get out there and just do it like the best athletes in the world!

I'm guessing your answers were Starbucks, Disney, Las Vegas, and Nike. That's the power of brands. They're shortcuts in your brain telling you how to think about a company or, as you're about to discover, about the dental practice.

Brand Examples

There are no "right" or "wrong" brands—just brands that connect your office with people who desire the quality and type of dentistry you want to provide. Here is a list of eleven possible practice brands. The first two examples speak directly to implant excellence. The others don't exclude implant excellence, and might be examples of brands that are more appropriate for your practice.

1. A high-end surgical and/or restorative practice that specializes in replacing missing teeth with implants.
2. A family practice that will do your implants right in our office—no referral needed.
3. A cosmetic office that will change your smile and change your life.
4. A dental spa that will change the way the world looks at you—and the way you look at the world.
5. A dental center that provides you world-class dentistry—right here in our small town.
6. An office where you can receive high-quality restorative dentistry *and* a beautiful smile.

7. A neighborhood practice that is open at convenient times where you can have all of your dentistry done under one roof.
8. A dental office that is full of friendly people who will take exceptional care of your entire family.
9. A practice where your fears will vanish as you gently receive the dentistry you need.
10. A clinic where you can have all that dentistry you've been putting off for years done while you snooze.
11. A dental center that will accept your insurance plan and provide dentistry at a reasonable cost.

Even though your brand is contained in other people's heads, it's an extension of *who* you are, *what* you do, and *how* you do it. With enough repetitions, your brand becomes words, images, and emotions in other people's minds. Contrary to popular opinion, brands are not names, logos, slogans, advertisements, and tag lines fabricated by some New York ad agency—although these may be the bridges from your office to the public's mind. Brands must be based on rock-solid *who's, what's,* and *how's.*

What's Your Brand?

If your brand is something along the lines of, "A dental office that is pretty much like all the other dental offices in the area," you're a commodity. If you're in the commodity business, it will severely limit your high-end practice branding options. Or is your brand something more specific that forms a bridge with the deeply held desires of a specific group of people? I hope so.

In your journal or notebook, write what you believe your brand is right now. Don't sugarcoat your answer. You will have a chance to enhance your answer in a minute.

Next, create what you would like your brand to be. In your journal or notebook, write the words, images, and emotions you would like to see in other people's heads concerning your dental practice. Then, write a brand definition using the ones above as examples. Follow these three guidelines:

1. Define your brand with only one sentence.
2. Begin your definition with "A _____ that/where…."
3. The words "you" or "your" must appear in the brand statement. The brand definition must connect with a deeply-held desire that your potential patients have.

Your continual challenge is moving from where you are now to where you want to be by changing *who* you are, *what* you do, and *how* you do it. You've already discovered how to enhance *who* you are by focusing on your character. In the coming chapters, you will learn numerous methods to improve *what* you do and *how* you do it. When you discover a method that resonates with you, immediately write it in your journal or notebook along with a plan for implementing the method.

Brand Stories

Companies that are powerful brands have huge collections of stories which dramatize the words, images, and emotions of their brands. Southwest Airlines has thousands of stories about employees who gave fun-loving service to their flyers. Many of Nike's commercials dramatize the stories of athletes who have excelled while wearing Nike shoes.

You need to collect brand stories of people who have benefited from your implant dentistry. These stories then can be told to your community with marketing and public relations. You will learn how to be a master marketer in Step 2.

It's also a wonderful idea to amass stories about times when your team members delivered top-notch service to patients. Keep these stories alive by repeating them often. This will help you create an office culture that is a walking example of your brand.

> *Brands are the stories that unite us all*
> *in a common purpose within an enterprise,*
> *and connect us with the people we serve on the outside.*
> *These brand stories give meaning to who we are*
> *and what we do.*
>
> MARK THOMSON

Branding as a Recruiting Tool

Properly presented, your brand is a powerful recruiting tool. It should be so compelling and pervasive that you have a waiting list of people who want to work for you. In your area, the front office people, hygienists, and clinical assistants talk amongst themselves. They know which dental practices differentiate themselves, what the differentiation is, and for which practices they would be a good match. In addition, the hiring messages you use should be targeted toward the people who will exemplify your brand, fit in with your positive attitude team, and be a walking billboard for your practice.

Practice Differentiation

Every morning on his way to work, a factory foreman passed a shop selling clocks. He always stopped in front of the shop, looked at the biggest clock in the shop, adjusted the time on his wrist watch, and proceeded to work. He did this every day for years. The shop owner noticed and became very curious. Finally one day he stopped the man and asked him what he was doing. The man told the shop owner he was the foreman of the factory down the street, and every day it was his duty to blow the end-of-the-day whistle at 5 pm. The shop owner started laughing. He said, "Everyday at 5 pm, when the factory whistle blows, I use it to adjust the time on the clocks in my shop."

This story teaches us two very important lessons. First, don't copy what average dentists are doing in your area. It will lead to everybody doing what everybody else is doing—a sure prescription for mediocrity. Second, if you model others, only select people who you know are successfully doing what you would like to accomplish. Don't limit your model search to your local area: outstanding practices can be anywhere in the world.

If you don't differentiate your practice, then you're a commodity and have no unique brand, and who in your area is going to be attracted to you? Certainly not people who share your values, because they don't know what your values are. If you're a commodity, people will think you're just like all those other dentists and come to you for all the wrong reasons—like, "You were on the insurance list," or "Your office was close to my home."

If you're just like everybody else, your fees will need to be just like everybody else's. Once you're in the commodity trap, it's a challenge to escape. But it can be done with the right strategy.

Conclusion

I hope you see that branding is way more than a flashy ad or a memorable jingle. Your brand is a dramatic declaration of who you are, what you do, and how you do it. That declaration is beneficial to you. It will be the standard that you will have to live up to. Brand You will make it easier for you to locate and select appropriate team members.

In addition, your brand will be beneficial to the team. It will remind them of what they need to do and how they need to do it. Brand You will be beneficial to your community. It will be the bridge though which they find a dental office that gives them what they uniquely desire in the way they desire it. With effective branding, everyone wins.

Henry Ford said, "You can't build a reputation on what you're *going* to do." You build a reputation on what you actually do. Doing is what the next four steps to implant excellence are all about. The next step is to be a master marketer. It's vital that you keep reading because having an excellent implant practice without marketing is like winking at a person in the dark. You know what you're doing, but nobody else does.

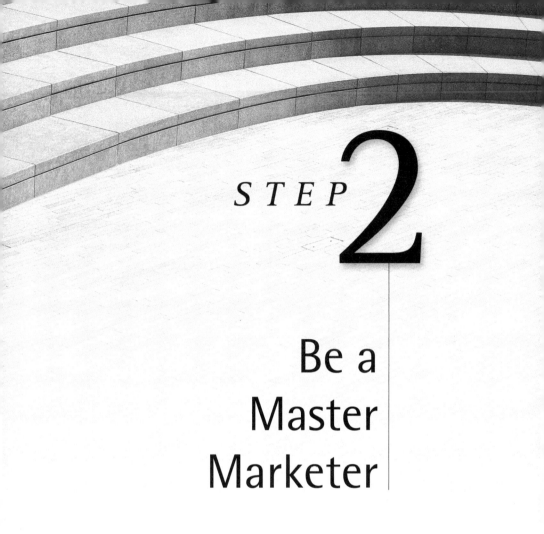

STEP 2

Be a Master Marketer

NOW THAT YOU'VE BUILT THE SOLID FOUNDATION for a great dental practice, you need to discover how to attract the customers who desire the quality of dentistry you want to provide. If you don't do an effective job of attracting these people, moving toward implant excellence will always be a struggle. When these people willingly walk through your door, advancing toward your dream practice will be a pleasure.

How Apple Does It

I'm a huge fan of the way Apple markets their products and services. Sure, they have terrific products with outstanding styling. But it's Apple's marketing that allows them to sell their merchandize for double the price of their competition. Here are six ways they do it:

1. **Turn Ordinary into Extraordinary:** Dell doesn't make bad products. They make ordinary products. Dell has 108,000 employees. Their 2012 revenue was $57 billion, and their market cap was $25 billion. Apple makes extraordinary products and provides extraordinary services like iTunes. They have 50,000 employees. They sold $156 billion in products and services in 2012 and have a market cap of $417 billion. Apple's market cap went up over $9 billion the day I wrote this paragraph! In your own small way, you can do the same in your community by turning your "ordinary" practice into an extraordinary one by providing outstanding dental implant services.

2. **Justify Your Price:** Don't try to win the "race to the bottom" on price. Apple certainly doesn't. There will also be someone willing to lower their fees more than you. Instead, justify your fees with your advanced training, skill, quality and caring.

3. **Communicate in an Audience-Friendly Way:** Ever closely studied Apple's ads? They aren't loaded boring facts and statistics. The ads focus on how you will look and feel using their products. Many dentists communicate in logical ways that appeal to themselves and other dentists. Instead of communicating to impress, you should communicate to influence.

4. **Extend the Experience:** An interesting new word has popped up in the English language – unboxing. To really understand what is means, go to YouTube and check out people's videos of them opening Apple boxes to see their bright, shiney, new, products for the first time. Apple designs their boxes to match the elegant design of the products inside to extend the experience. Do the same in your office. Wrap outstanding patient experiences around your outstanding dental care.

5. **Build a Tribe:** Ever tried talking your teenager into purchasing a full-featured smart phone instead of buying a $200 iPhone? Good luck. To them, an owning an iPhone is a badge of honor that identifies them as a member of the Apple tribe. Does your office have a tribe of loyal followers that would only come to you and recommend you to all of their family and friends? If not, follow the advice in this book to create one.

6. **Become "The Name":** You don't buy tissues. You buy Kleenex. Likewise, people don't buy MP3 players. They buy iPods. There are two ways to be "The Name": 1) Be there first in your marketplace, or 2) Be so much better and/or unique than the competition that you clearly stand out. Apple isn't always the first. They are almost always the best and the most unique. You need to do the same.

People Have Varying Desires for Implant Dentistry

Let's quantify people on a +10 to −10 scale. People you consider +10 patients come to your office asking for quality implant dentistry. Their pockets are stuffed full of $100 bills. You present your recommendations, and they immediately ask, "When can we get started!?"

People you think of as +7 patients don't come in the door asking for implant dentistry, but after you have a series of conversations with them they readily agree to act on your recommendations. Money, time, and trust aren't problems for these people.

Those you rate as +4 people don't come in the door asking for implant dentistry. After you have your implant dentistry conversations, they have to think about it for a while before beginning. Money may be a challenge for them. As a result, they may have to finance their care.

Patients you deem 0 may take years to have their implant dentistry completed. As it isn't a high priority for them *and* finances are a big challenge, they may have to wait for the time to be right to proceed. For example, they may say, "We need to wait until the kids graduate from college."

People you regard as −4 patients *may* complete their implant dentistry, but only if the time is right *and* their situation becomes desperate.

The patients you rate at −7 or below would never have implants. These last three types of patients (0, −4, −7) may end up in your recare system.

Where Do You Set the Bar?

Some dental offices specialize in dental implants, have wonderful reputations in their communities, and position themselves to attract +10 people. Some offices are high-end general practices with excellent reputations, performing numerous implants and attracting patients rated +4 and higher. Many offices are high-quality family practices that perform a few implants and attract people 4 and higher. Most offices are high-volume clinics that don't undertake implants and attract people from −4 to −10.

I'm not here to tell you what kind of practice you should have and what type of people you should aim to attract. You already decided that for yourself in chapter 1. I am here to encourage you to be your own marketing expert and create a marketing plan to attract the people you desire, however high or low they may be rated. Chapter 5 will be your Marketing 101 introduction.

Your Three Marketing Tools

Webster defines marketing as the process of promoting, selling, and distributing a product or service. In a dental office, that definition would equate to influencing people to walk in your door, gaining case acceptance, and performing clinical dentistry. Because many dentists don't want to view themselves as advertisers or salespeople, we typically segment and define dental marketing in three narrower, professionally "scrubbed" ways.

Internal Marketing is the process of making it easy for your current patients to accept more implant dentistry as well as using your current patients to help you attract new patients. As you will learn in Chapter 6, internal marketing has the advantages of being extremely effective and very low cost.

External Marketing is the process of *paying* the media to gain the attention of people so they seek out your services. External marketing can be expensive because it involves purchasing yellow page ads, newspaper and magazine print ads, direct mail, Internet marketing, radio and TV commercials, and alternative advertising such as airport signs and billboards. Chapter 7 will be your guide to extraordinary external marketing.

Public Relations is the process of *using* the media to gain the attention of non-patients so they call you on the phone for an appointment. Public relations can also include your office team members being active in the community (resulting in increased new patient flow), and working with other professional offices to increase referrals. In Chapter 8, you will discover several innovative ways to harness the power of public relations.

Chapter 9 will show you how to create a wow website that will be an important component of your internal marketing, external marketing, and public relations marketing plan.

But before you can explore or utilize the three types of marketing, it's important that you first learn to be your own marketing expert.

CHAPTER 5

Be Your Own Marketing Expert

I CAN'T TELL YOU the number of times I've seen dentists spend money on high-priced marketing that generates little or no business. To prevent this from happening, you or someone in your office needs to become a marketing expert. This doesn't mean you will design and execute your entire marketing plan; it means you know enough to make sure the outside marketing people attend to your best interests and produce measurable results.

Have the Product on the Shelf before You Begin Marketing

Lexus wouldn't advertise their LS460 if they didn't have the car in their showrooms. Doing so would be worse than not advertising at all, because consumers would discover that Lexus couldn't deliver on its advertised promises. The same is true with your practice. You must have the surgical and/or restorative implant skills to deliver the high-quality dentistry and the high-level service your brand is promising.

After nearly 20 years as an educator and academic clinician at the University of Miami, I retired and went into private practice. I used everything I knew (and thought I knew) to market the office. After making almost every mistake in the book, it dawned on me that my practice was turning into a very expensive hobby! So I read every marketing and self-help book I could lay my hands on. I attended numerous practice management and dental marketing seminars. Over a two-year period, I invested thousands of dollars and thousands of hours to become a marketing expert. And my hard work has paid off. I've now built a very successful private practice by providing quality implant dentistry to my patients.

I've also studied the offices of hundreds of my students. There were many commonalities and differences among the practices, but the factor with the most variety was marketing. One size does not fit all when it comes to dental marketing! Although there is no ideal program that can routinely be duplicated, there *is* one best marketing plan for you. In the four chapters that follow, you will discover some of the best ideas I unearthed as I learned marketing the hard way. I want you to learn it the easy way. This chapter will start the process by giving you eight keys that unlock the vault to dental marketing success.

Key #1: Don't Play It Safe

When it comes to marketing, don't play it safe by copying the methods of everyone else in your area. If you do, limited results and off-target patients will be your reward. Many dentists don't market at all or have very traditional marketing methods as a result of two unwritten rules they follow. The first unwritten rule says, "Dentists aren't supposed to advertise. That would be highly unprofessional." I don't agree with that at all. Who loses if you don't publicly promote your implant excellence? People in your community lose because they don't learn about the most recent advances in implant dentistry and your ability to deliver those innovations. Your team and you lose because you won't be able to receive the emotional and financial rewards that accompany the delivery of the highest quality dental care. Finally, our profession loses. When you raise the quality level of your practice and perform more top-notch dentistry, sooner or later other practices will see the light (or feel the heat) and improve the quality of their care, too.

The second unwritten rule says, "I'm in the same boat as the other dentists in my area. I can't rock the boat and upset my fellow sailors. They might get seasick and blame me. So I'm going to play it safe, keep my head down, and do what everybody else does—especially when it comes to something as visible as marketing." However, playing it safe is habit forming and leads to a life of mediocrity. How exciting is that?

> *Those who give up liberty to purchase a little safety deserve neither liberty nor safety.*
> BENJAMIN FRANKLIN

Key #2: Market Internally First

If your practice is like most, the best prospects for implant dentistry are your current patients. Give them the opportunity to say yes to the best. Mail letters and/or postcards to your existing patients. During their recare visits, have your hygienists communicate the recent advances in and advantages of implant dentistry. Give the patients logical and emotional reasons for taking action. Convey enthusiasm and make it affordable by providing investment options. And of course, take great care of your current patients so they enthusiastically refer friends and family.

Key #3: Begin with the End in Mind

John F. Kennedy began with the end in mind when he challenged the nation to put a man on the moon within a decade. Mary Kay Ash began with the end in mind when she started Mary Kay Cosmetics to give women opportunities outside of the traditional workplace. In the first chapter, you created the practice of your dreams. With that done, you can create your own marketing plan to attract the patients who are predisposed to accepting first-rate implant dentistry.

New patients are the lifeblood of an implant practice. When it comes to these people, there are three questions you need to ask:

1. How many implant cases do you need to complete each month to meet your dream practice financial goals?

2. At your present rate of case acceptance, how many new patients do you need to see each month to achieve the goal of question #1?

3. How many new patients each month can you comfortably take through the implant acceptance process, which includes a comprehensive exam, thorough diagnosis, development of a complete treatment plan, and a series of relaxed, face-to-face conversations?

The second and third questions address the number of new patients in your practice. The second question concerns finances. The third question concerns emotions and ethics. Both questions must have similar answers to create the financial and emotional/ethical goals of your dream practice. Here's an example of what I mean: Let's say you need to complete 16 implant cases a month to meet your dream practice's financial goals. Based on your current rate of case acceptance, to complete those 16 cases you would need to see 57 new patients per month (the answer to question #2). However, you believe that you could take only 32 new patients per month through the case acceptance process (the answer to question #3). The mismatch of numbers between questions 2 and 3 will force you to take one of two paths.

Path One. You cherry-pick through 57 new patients in a vain attempt to find 16 implant cases by doing rushed and incomplete exams, diagnoses, treatment plans, and case conversations. This approach will prevent you from achieving your financial goals because the kinds of people who desire comprehensive implant dentistry aren't attracted to rushed practices. In addition, people don't typically say yes to comprehensive dentistry in hurried situations. You will also fail to achieve your emotional goals because the entire team will be going nuts roller-skating from room to room with a 12-minute lunch and no breaks. I've even seen Path One doctors who didn't meet their financial goals try to fix the situation by seeing *more* new patients each month. This just makes matters worse because **going harder and faster down the wrong path gets you to where you don't want to go— quicker!**

Path Two. You enhance your marketing plan to attract 32 patients who are more inclined to say yes to implant dentistry, and/or improve your case communication process so a higher percentage of people accept comprehensive care. Do you see how this second path will lead to your financial **and** emotional goals as you provide the quality of care your patients deserve? I encourage you to take this path and base the number of new patients you see each month on your answer to the third question above.

Key # 4: Know Your Market Area

To construct an effective marketing campaign, it's vital that you know the demographics and psychographics of the people in your market area. Demographics measure the statistical data of a population group, especially the data showing average age, income, and education. The ideal implant patients you're looking for are over 55 years of age and have moderate to high incomes. Psychographics measure the attitudes, values, lifestyles, and opinions of the population group, usually for marketing purposes.

When it comes right down to it, all the population groups just want their missing teeth and denture problems solved, but different population groups tend to value the benefits of implant dentistry differently. Here are four groups of people who are likely candidates for implants and a list of the benefits each group desires. The information is based on the Values and Lifestyle Survey done by the Stanford Research Institute.

1. **Belongers.** As the name implies, these people like to be identified with and belong to a larger group. They could be Midwesterners who drive Fords and Chevys because they are proud Americans whose cars are American-made, or they could be part of a close-knit ethnic group. Enduring relationships are valued extremely highly by belongers. Ideally, they want you to be part of their group. If you are, they will tend to do business with you and listen to your recommendations. If you're not part of their group, it may take some time to gain their trust; but once you do, you're in. Belongers can be any age, and don't want anything too fancy. They just want something that works well and is reasonably priced.

Belongers like marketing that emphasizes relationships and stability, like the State Farm Insurance "Like a Good Neighbor State Farm Is There" TV ads, or a tag line after a business name that declares, "Serving the Community for Over Thirty Years." When you market to belongers, make it obvious that you're a local dentist and a trusted member of the community. When belongers are in your office, take the time to gain their trust and rapport and don't pressure them to accept implant dentistry.

2. **Emulators.** These people desperately desire to look good and be successful in business. They wear fashionable clothes and go to trendy bars and restaurants. Emulators would love to own a brand-new BMW 7 Series car, but all they can afford right now is a 3 Series on an affordable lease plan. Emulators don't have a lot of money yet, but they will spend or borrow it to purchase products and services that make them look successful and sexy.

   Emulators are attracted to marketing with photos of young, sexy, and successful people. When emulators with missing teeth are in your office, ask them, "How important is it for you to have an attractive smile?" They will invariably answer, "A lot!" Then show them how implant dentistry will give them the most attractive smile possible.

3. **Achievers.** Emulators aspire to be achievers. Emulators *want* to be successful. Achievers *are* successful. Emulators *want* a lot of money. Achievers *have* a lot of money. Achievers own Lexus, Mercedes, BMW, or Cadillac automobiles. Now that achievers are successful and have the financial resources, they want to spend it on the best products and services.

   Achievers are attracted to marketing that shows you are the best dentist who provides the highest quality dentistry. When achievers with missing teeth are in your office, communicate how implant dentistry is the best care available.

4. **Socially Conscious.** These people tend to be highly educated, and because they want to make "planet earth" a better place to live, they are "green" oriented. The socially conscious use public transportation or drive Volvos, VWs, or Honda/Toyota hybrids. Socially conscious

people place a high value on health and would never have a mercury-infested amalgam filling in their mouths. They want to make the intelligent decision when it comes to products and services.

Socially conscious people are attracted to marketing that is intelligent. No hype. No free offers. When socially conscious people are in your office, stress the intelligent benefits of implants and educate them about what you do.

Key #5: Create a Budget

Your marketing expenditures can easily get away from you if you don't set and abide by a budget. In most of the offices I've worked with, the yearly marketing budget is 5 percent of the practice's gross from the previous 12 months. This means the marketing budget for $1 million practice would be from $30,000 to $50,000 per year. For implant practices, however, it should be 5–10%. It's not necessary to spend equal amounts of money each month, however. You may save by purchasing several ads at the same time, for instance, and then those ads would run at regular intervals throughout the year.

Key #6: Use a Variety of Marketing Methods

About four years ago, a dentist attending one of my *Implant Seminars Courses* told me a very interesting and revealing story. He had a new patient come in and say, "I received your mailing six months ago (external marketing). I read the article about you four weeks ago (public relations). I just talked to a patient of yours who said you're a terrific dentist (internal marketing). That was the third time in six months I've heard about your practice. Now I feel good about coming in to see you." Isn't that interesting? This person needed three exposures from three different sources to make the decision to schedule a visit. That's why it's so important to create a marketing campaign that includes a variety of the internal marketing, external marketing, and public relations methods that you will learn in the next few chapters.

Key #7: Be Consistent and Persistent

You need to be persistent with your internal marketing, external marketing, and public relations. Many dentists make the mistake of quickly jumping from one marketing method to another. It takes time for most forms of marketing to show results. You need to be consistent with your marketing in two ways:

1. Make sure all your marketing messages consistently and accurately communicate your brand. More than one brand message just confuses people.

2. Be consistent with the targeting of your marketing plan. Know the demographics and psychographics of your market area and direct your appeal to the group(s) most likely to want implant dentistry. When you try to appeal to everyone, you appeal to no one.

Key #8: Track Your Marketing

It's important to think like a business person and track your marketing efforts. When people schedule initial visits on the phone, ask them, "How did you find out about us?" Make the question part of your first phone call script. One word of caution here: people can't always remember exactly why they called *you*. Maybe one marketing method brought your practice into their awareness and another form of marketing sparked them to pick up the phone and call. Both forms were important, but they will only remember the second. Accept the fact that sometimes you're not going to know exactly what's working. That may be okay as long as the entire marketing plan is effective. One attractive feature of internet marketing is that it is highly measurable.

> *Half the money I spend on advertising is wasted.*
> *The trouble is I don't know which half.*
>
> JOHN WANAMAKER

Conclusion

In this chapter, you discovered why it's so important for you or someone else in your office to be a marketing expert. The next four chapters will give you some powerful internal marketing, external marketing, public relations, and website ideas.

Carl Frederick said, "The key to your universe is that you can choose." It will be up to you to choose the ideas you believe will work best for your practice, in your area, to attract the people who will be the future patients in the practice of your dreams.

CHAPTER 6
Intriguing Internal Marketing

THE FOUNDER AND FIRST PRESIDENT OF TEMPLE UNIVERSITY, Russell H. Conwell, gave his "Acres of Diamonds" presentation over 6,000 times to audiences around the world. The featured story in the presentation described a farmer who heard of the riches that could be had by prospecting for diamonds. So he sold his farm, said goodbye to the family, packed his gear, and went to make his fortune. After years of world travel and gemless digging, he became disheartened and committed suicide.

Meanwhile, back at his farm, the new owner noticed a shiny object in a stream running through the property. It was a diamond of enormous value—the first of many to be found on the land. The farm was literally covered with acres of diamonds.

Your dental practice is like the farm, and you are like the first farmer and simply haven't noticed the diamonds in your own back yard—your existing patients who are candidates for implant dentistry. The moral of the story is to look for people who need implants within your practice first, using internal marketing. *Then* look outside your practice.

There are two aspects of internal marketing we will explore: (1) make it easy for your current patients to accept implant dentistry, and (2) work with your current patients to attract new ones.

Make It Easy for Your Current Patients to Accept Implant Dentistry

In J.K. Rowling's *Harry Potter* series, one of her most ingenious inventions is the Invisibility Cloak. Harry and his friends place the cloak over themselves and become invisible. They can see and hear outsiders—but they can't be seen. You may be unaware that you're throwing the Invisibility Cloak over your practice, but that's exactly what happens when you fail to maintain frequent contact with your current patients to nurture your relationship. Here are some symptoms of YOICS—Your Office Invisibility Cloak Syndrome:

- holes mysteriously appear in the hygiene schedule
- new patient flow drops off
- case acceptance is lower than normal
- increasing numbers of recare patients are past due
- production either levels off or declines

The YOICS Cure

The cure for YOICS is simple: stay in frequent contact with your patients. Here are two ways to regularly communicate with them.

1. **Use a patient messaging software system** that provides a secure and effective way for your office to directly communicate with patients by automatically sending personalized, real-time text messages to their mobile phones, e-mail addresses, and/or pagers. The system integrates with almost every practice management software system so there is no need for double entry. You can also send customized newsletters, birthday greetings, recare reminders, and more.

2. **Send a letter to your denture patients.** Send a version of the following sample letter to all your former denture patients. This is especially important because they may not come to the office for recare appointments as often as non-denture patients.

SAMPLE LETTER

Gentle, State of the Art Dental Implant Care for Mature Adults

We invite you to return to our office and become part of a special dental care program for mature adults ages 50 and over.

You may be saying to yourself, "I've never heard of a dental practice having a special program for the 50+ age group."

You're correct. It is uncommon. Over the past few years, I realized that I thoroughly enjoy working with mature people who appreciate the importance of excellent oral health and the improved quality of life it brings. As a result, I've shifted a portion of my practice to address the special needs of the 50+ age group.

Dental Needs for People over 50 Are Quite Different from People Who Are 35.

With time, teeth discolor, wear down and may even be lost. To replace their missing teeth, some people wear dentures, which can be a real hassle. Wearing dentures speeds the loss of bone that supports the dentures. This is why dentures (especially lower ones) loosen with time. The result can be eating and speech problems, gagging and even displacement of the denture. Adhesives may help only a little or not
at all.

Solving the above problems require special skills ... skills that my staff and I are qualified and eager to provide you.

At the Center for Complete Dentistry, we offer advanced dental implant services.

Are you a candidate for dental implants? To find out, please answer the following questions:

- Do you take your lower denture out during the day?
- Do you never wear your lower denture?
- Do you have speech difficulties while wearing your lower denture?
- Does your lower denture move excessively?

(Continued on reverse.)

- Do you avoid certain foods because of your lower denture?
- Do you eat better without your lower denture in place?
- Do you have less chewing ability with your dentures than you had with your partial denture or natural teeth?
- Are you unhappy with the size, shape or fit of your lower denture?

If you answered, "Yes," to **any** of the above questions, please call 954-455-3434 to schedule an evaluation for the most advanced, gentle and specialized dental implant care available. In addition, we offer payment plans that fit your budget.

We're just minutes from your home.

The Center for Complete Dentistry is conveniently located at 1920 E. Hallandale Beach Blvd., Suite 800.

So please come back and visit us. Enjoy a cup of coffee, tea or fruit juice on us. Our juice bar is always stocked; and one of the staff will be happy to serve you. I'm confident you will enjoy your visit. We look forward to seeing you again soon.

Warmest regards,

Donald Lambert

Donald Lambert, DDS

**To learn more, visit www.CenterForCompleteDentistry.com.
Don't wait a day longer.
You have nothing to lose except your problems.**

In-Office Communications with Current Patients

The best way to make it easy for your current patients to accept implant dentistry is to communicate with them while they're already in the office. Here are six effective ways to connect with them:

1. On a table in your reception area, have a photo album showing before and after photos of your implant patients. It's nice to have the patients' testimonials next to their photos. My Publisher is an excellent place to obtain the software and materials to make an album with impact. The download is free at www.mypublisher.com.

2. On your office walls, hang *professionally* done, smiling photos of your patients after their dentistry has been completed. Have photos of the different types of implant cases you routinely do.

3. When it comes to implants, it's vitally important that your entire team knows what you do, why you do it, and the results you achieve. To accomplish this, at a series of team meetings, show the team the ImplantVision narrated software animations. Then present a few implant cases you've completed. With each case, exhibit all the patient records and discuss the factors leading to your diagnosis and treatment. Now show them the records for an implant case you've completed and ask how they would diagnose and treat the patient. Everyone on your team needs this information because people in and out of the office will ask them about implant dentistry.

4. At recare visits, have your hygienists ask the patients, "Have you heard or read about a dental topic you would like to know more about?" It's always better if patients bring up a topic first. If they do, the hygienists can discuss the topic during the visit. Incidentally, once hygienists pick up perio instruments, they go to Perio Land. And when they're in Perio Land, they don't come out until the visit is over. Moral: hygienists should discuss non-hygiene topics at the beginning of recare visits.

5. Show patients educational materials on a variety of implant topics. A picture is worth a thousand words, and a well-done DVD is worth ten thousand words.

6. If the patients ask about implants or mention problems that may be related to missing teeth, or if your hygienists see opportunities for implants, make it easy for patients to take the first steps toward having implants with the following conversation: "Tom, I'm glad you mentioned your jaw joints are clicking. Those two missing teeth on your lower right side may be causing your jaw joint on the right side to not receive the support it needs. Can you see on the TV monitor that the upper teeth above the space are coming down farther than they should? The missing teeth are also causing you to use your other teeth more than necessary.

   "Also, take a look in the mirror. Do you see where your right cheek is a little bit into the space where the teeth should be? There are several ways of replacing missing teeth. The doctor usually recommends implants for cases like yours. Let's take a look at this short video on lower implants and why they may be the best choice.

   "Do you have any questions about implants so far?"

   If they don't have questions, answer "Great. Would you like to explore the possibility of having implants? We can talk to Dr. Starck about it when she comes in to do her exam."

   If they do have questions, answer them and proceed with the "Would you like to explore the possibility of" question.

   When you come in, the hygienist should do this handoff: "Dr. Starck, Tom has some clicking in his jaw joints which may be due to his two missing teeth on the right side. We've briefly discussed implants, and Tom has seen the implant video. He's seen how the upper teeth above the space are coming down farther than they should. We also talked about why the missing teeth may be causing problems with his other teeth and how his jaw joint on the right side probably isn't getting the support it needs. Tom has seen how his right cheek is collapsing a little bit into the space where the teeth should be. I told Tom that you typically suggest implants in cases like his and will take a look and tell us what you think."

This type of handoff accomplishes two goals: It gives you the information you need to take the next step, and it allows Tom to hear his implant story for a second time.

Work with Current Patients to Attract New Ones

The second way you can market internally is to work with your current patients to attract new ones. First, you need to gain their loyalty. Then you can make it easy for them to refer their family and friends.

If a $75,000 piece of equipment was missing from your practice tomorrow morning, how concerned would you be? How hard would you work to recover it? What steps would you take to make sure it wouldn't be lost again? I'm betting you would be tremendously concerned; you wouldn't stop looking until you found it; and you would make certain it never happened again.

I have an important follow-up question for you: Would you take the same steps if you lost one loyal patient? I hope so, because their value is way more than $75,000.

There are four levels of patients you can have in your practice:

Level One: Loyal. "My experience far exceeds my expectations."

Level Two: Satisfied. "My experience meets my expectations."

Level Three: Apathetic. "My experience is a little short of my expectations."

Level Four: Unhappy. "My experience falls way short of my expectations."

Unhappy patients usually leave your practice as soon as possible. **Apathetic** patients tend to move on when something better comes along. They may switch to an office that opens closer to their home. **Satisfied** patients will stay with you until a significant change occurs, such as the way you deal with insurance, a noticeable fee increase, or if they (or you) move out of the area. **Loyal** patients are with you for life. If they move 1,500 miles away, loyal patients will fly back for their visits. Loyal patients create positive word-of-mouth advertising for you and refer family, friends, and total strangers to you. In addition, loyal patients and loyal team members are connected in a self-perpetuating cycle that creates great dental offices. The cycle looks like this:

- You have an office full of **loyal patients**
- who complete comprehensive care and refer numerous family and friends with personalities similar to themselves
- which significantly improves your net profit
- that allows you to attract, train, and maintain the best people
- which creates a **loyal team**
- which delivers five-star patient care and builds close patient relationships
- which keeps and attracts more **loyal patients**
- and the loyalty cycle rolls on and on.

The Loyalty Cycle

Loyal Patients

who complete comprehensive care and refer others

which improves your net profit

that allows you to attract, train, and maintain the best people

which creates a

Loyal Team

who deliver five-star patient care

which attracts and keeps

Walking Billboards

Loyal patients are walking billboards for your practice. It's interesting—and revealing—to calculate how much each loyal patient is worth to your practice over an 11-year period. Here's how to do it:

1. Calculate, on average, how much money one loyal patient spends in your practice over an 11-year period. Remember, the person probably spends way more than your average patients, especially during the first year. As an example, a loyal patient spends $9,000 the first year and an average of $800 per year for the next 10 years. The total for 11 years is $17,000.

2. How many new patients does the average loyal patient refer to your office each year? As an example, your average loyal patient refers four people per year to you.

3. Multiply your answer to the second question by 11, as the average walking billboard will be a patient in your office for around 11 years. In our example, the walking billboard will refer 44 people.

4. Multiply the number you calculated in the third question by the total fees each referred person pays over 11 years. As an example, the average referred person spends $5,000 the first year and $800 per year over the next 10 years, for a total expenditure of $13,000. $13,000 times 44 (how many people are spending the same amount with you) equals $572,000.

5. Add together the figures you calculated in the first and fourth questions. In our example, the total would be $589,000! And that figure doesn't include the number of people who would be referred by the 44 original referees.

What number did you come up with? When I speak to dental groups, most dentists tell me numbers in the $400,000 to $2,000,000 range. So here's my question to you. If each loyal patient in your practice is worth $589,000, what would you do to attract, nurture, and retain that person? Would you take them and their spouse out to dinner every couple of years, or provide some other type of referral gift? How would you and your team greet them at their recare visits?

The Loyalty Exercise

The best way to create patient loyalty is to focus on loyalty, not on satisfaction (which is what most dental offices do). You can create an excellent team meeting by presenting the loyalty information earlier in this chapter. Then do the five-step calculation outlined on the previous page. Next, ask the loyalty question "How can we treat people so they become loyal patients and are *compelled* to tell their friends and family and strangers on the street how great we are?" Finally, have your team come up with five to 10 answers and a plan to implement each approach.

Make It Easy for Them to Refer Their Family and Friends

Now that you've gained your patients' loyalty, it's time to take the next step and make it easy for them to refer their family and friends. I'm not a fan of pressuring patients to do things. I *am* an advocate of removing resistances so people comfortably take the actions that improve their lives.

Some dental consultants teach techniques for requesting patient referrals that I think are too pushy. The techniques require team members to ask questions at contrived times and put pressure on patients to give answers. Here's an example of what I mean: "John, I hope you like your new implants and over-denture. Do you have any family or friends who might benefit from the same dentistry?" I prefer waiting for naturally-occurring times and making offers to help. Here are two examples of what I mean:

1. John comments on how much he likes her new over-denture. Your team member or you respond, "John, I'm so glad you like it. If you have any family or friends who would benefit from this kind of care, we would be glad to schedule them a complimentary visit. You can even come with them the first time if you'd like."

2. John comments on how much he likes coming to your office. Your team member or you respond, "John, I'm so glad you like coming to our office. If you have any family or friends who would benefit from our care, we would be glad to schedule them a complimentary visit. You can even come with them the first time if you'd like."

Of course, the family and friends can come to the office without your current patient. You will learn how to do this complimentary—and effective—meet-and-greet visit in Chapter 11.

The above two examples occur at times chosen by the patients and don't require patients to answer. You may be thinking, "What if our patients never mention how much they love our clinical care or us?" If that's the case, look in the mirror. Maybe it's you! You receive referrals by *earning* them, not by asking for them.

Referral Gifts

The best referral gift you can give a patient is a heartfelt thank you in person, on a phone call, or with a handwritten note. If you do give gifts that cost money, be absolutely certain to do something to make the gift more personal. Don't just send a gift certificate to a restaurant. Insert the gift certificate inside a handwritten thank you note. Or, in the case of extremely loyal patients, take them and their spouses/friends to dinner, on your tab.

I encourage you *not* to make each successive gift more expensive as the number of referrals increases. After the 25th referral, they'll think, "Where's my BMW?" Mix up your referral gifts—a written thank you, then a phone call, then some flowers, then a thank you in person, then tickets to the movies, etc.

The Power of "And"

As you've learned, creating and maintaining loyalty in your patients and team is the right thing to do, **and** it's good business. Through my life experiences, I discovered that's always the case. I've noticed some people go through life with a "but" mentality. As an example, "I can be an honest and ethical person, **but** I can't be as successful in business that way." "I can provide better compensation for my team, **but** I would net less." I'm encouraging you to get off your **but** and get on your **and**. The word "and" is additive: everyone comes out ahead. Life is not a zero sum game where you lose if I win and vice versa. Life done right is additive, and win-win situations abound.

Who wins when you purchase this book? You win because the book helps you create implant excellence. Your patients win because they receive better care.

Your team wins because they experience the joy of doing more comprehensive, throw-away-the-roller-skates dentistry. I win because you're exposed to my philosophies and may want to attend our programs. Our profession wins because the level of care in your community will rise, and a rising tide lifts all the boats.

Conclusion

The next chapter will give you a zoo-full of examples on how to effectively market your practice externally. Read on.

CHAPTER 7

Extraordinary External Marketing

AFTER YOU CREATE AND IMPLEMENT an implant excellence internal marketing campaign, it's time to look externally and attract a select group of people who are not currently in your practice—people who have pains that implant dentistry can alleviate. To attract these people, you need the clinical skills and the non-clinical skills of marketing, practice management, and case acceptance that are specific to implant dentistry. In this chapter, you will learn the basics of external marketing. Depending on your unique practice characteristics, professional goals, and market area, you can use these basics as a starting point to create an effective external marketing program.

Implant Patients Want Solutions to their Problems

Suffering from missing teeth and/or wearing dentures are the ultimate dental disabilities. This puts you in a unique position when it comes to marketing your services as these people are keenly interested in the solutions that will alleviate the problems caused by their disabilities.

To reach these people, you must create a compelling advertising message and place it in the correct media location for your market area. While the same message can work almost everywhere, the advertising media, costs, and frequencies required vary tremendously based on your competition and market size. **There are no cookie-cutter solutions for creating the best external marketing campaign.** There are, however, *guidelines* you can use to create your ideal external marketing campaign.

Create Effective Problem/Solution Advertisements

All effective problem/solution ads have the same five components.

#1: Compelling Headlines

Headlines are the most important part of an ad. Every ad needs a headline, whether the medium is newspaper, magazine, radio, TV, the Internet, yellow pages, or direct mail. You'd be amazed at how many advertisers (dentists included) ignore this crucial requirement and spend fortunes on ads that don't produce.

#2: Present Problems and Offer Solutions

Your implant marketing should always send problem/solution messages. The basic template for your implant ads should be, "You have a serious problem (missing teeth or denture disabilities). If you don't do anything about the problem, it will only get worse and more painful. But fear not. We can fix it and have you looking like new with our advanced implant skills and techniques. See us before it's too late."

People will do more to avoid pain than to gain pleasure. In your ads, motivate them to action with *pain*, AND give them a direction to move toward with *pleasure*.

#3: Make Offers with Deadlines

The best ads make offers with deadlines asking consumers to take specific actions, such as making a phone call, attending an implant information meeting, or going to a website for a free report. Too many dental ads are just awareness ads not asking consumers to do anything. Think action, not awareness.

#4: Start the Pre-Qualifying Process

Problem/solution ads are the first step in your patient pre-qualifying process. These ads allow you to put screening steps in place to keep most unqualified patients from calling your office. In effect, your ad should say, "Only people with missing teeth or denture disabilities should respond to this ad."

#5: Track Responses

Track responses from a specific ad in a specific advertising medium to maximize the ROI (return on investment) of your advertising dollars. When you track results, you know where to best spend your advertising dollars in the future. Tracking can be done with a dedicated response phone number for a specific ad or phone numbers having extensions linked to specific ads.

In a nutshell, successful implant marketing is the process of creating the best ad headline and problem/solution message you can, placing the ad where you think it will have the most effectiveness (a 55+ demographic) and tracking its performance. Then continue this cycle until achieving your desired results.

Use Mass Media to Convey Your Message

You've created your problem/solution ad with the five components outlined above. To find enough patients who have problems that are solvable with your implant care, you must use mass media. Statistics show that only about 5 percent of people with missing teeth or denture disabilities will take action to receive implant dentistry. As a result of this low percentage, you must use mass media to communicate with an extremely large pool of potential patients with your problem/solution ads. In many ways, it's like finding a golden needle in a haystack. Mass media includes the "big four" traditional media (newspapers, glossy magazines, radio, and TV) as well as nontraditional media (the Internet, yellow pages, and direct mail).

Market Size

The size of your market area will heavily influence your external advertising decisions. In **smaller markets,** there's typically a scarcity of dental implant advertising. As a result, there's a large group of people waiting to hear solutions for their missing teeth and poorly fitting dentures.

Because the demographics of smaller markets are more homogeneous, the advertising media has fewer players and potential patients are easier to reach. The traditional media often dominate these markets, which makes any kind of media advertising a great choice. The Internet is poplular everywhere and should also be used. The small-market dentists who harness the power of the Internet early can enjoy an insurmountable lead over their competition.

Because of lower ad rates, it's possible to use all four of the traditional media to own the implant segment of dentistry in a small market

In **mid-sized markets**, the best medium could be any one of the big four. Because of higher costs, it's likely that you will use one or two of the four traditional mass media (newspapers, glossy magazines, radio, and TV). The Internet is a bigger factor in medium-sized markets, so your marketing plan should include it.

In **larger markets**, the risk increases for making mistakes and wasting incredible amounts of money. It's likely that only one form of traditional mass media will be in your budget. Your additional marketing will use the nontraditional forms. Effective marketing in the right media will generate excellent results, but you have to be far more careful about your strategies.

In larger markets, having an effective website using direct response principles needs to be on the top of your priority list. Only 1 percent of dental practice sites are designed in this way which will give you a major advantage in this area.

Traditional Media

The big four traditional media include newspapers, glossy magazines, radio, and TV. Even though they're oldies, they can still be goodies.

Newspapers

Newspapers have the least expensive cost per thousand views of all media. They also have longevity, which means ads can be clipped and saved—something that's not possible with radio and TV. For all their benefits newspapers are a changing medium. The bad news is that the cost per 1,000 customer views is going up. The good news is that people in the 55+ age group you're coveting are the ones still reading newspapers. Do you live in a small town? Congratulations. Small town people love their local newspaper!

Glossy Magazines

Because most glossy local magazines emphasize image versus health and comfort, they are a natural for cosmetic dentistry. But they can be big money drainers for implants if you don't know what you're doing. When you create a problem/solution ad as described earlier, your ads can be effective.

Radio

Radio still works well in the right markets. The way to find out if your market is one of them is by asking for the 55+ Tap Scan Reports for the stations you're considering. If these reports show the 55+ group is primarily listening to one or two local stations and the ad expense fits into your budget, radio may still work well for you.

Another option to consider is hosting your own once-a-week or once-a-month radio show. If you have the right personality and the time, this is an excellent strategy to make you the ultimate dental expert in your area.

Television

A properly scripted TV ad can generate a massive response. This means your screening systems are extremely important since the number of potential patients calling can be overwhelming. Almost all of your responses will come from people who aren't pre-qualified to financially commit to implants. Imagine having 50 to 100 phone calls every time a TV spot runs when only 5 percent of the callers will eventually accept your implant treatment plans. There is no way to handle the screening process in person without overwhelming your team.

Nontraditional Media: Internet

About 25-50 percent of your marketing budget should be spent on internet marketing.

There are two areas search engine marketing you should focus on:

1. **Search Engine Optimization (SEO):** SEO the process of affecting the visibility of a website or a web page in a search engine's "natural" or unpaid search results. In general, the earlier and more frequently a site appears in the search results list, the more visitors it will receive from the search engine's users. As an example, when people search for an implant dentist in Tulsa, OK, they will use key words such as "Tulsa implant dentist" or "dental implants Tulsa" or "implant dentistry Tulsa." These key words should be used in the headings and copy on the page or pages you devote to implants in your website. Remember, search engines want to make it easy for their users to find the information they desire. The search engines have become very adept at doing this. Are you just as good at being the website they direct their users to? Many website designers have more skills in design than marketing. I'm not saying design isn't important, but marketing is vital.

2. **Pay Per Click (PPC):** PPC is an internet advertising model used to direct traffic to websites, where advertisers pay when the ad is clicked. With search engines, advertisers typically bid on keyword phrases relevant to their target market. Content sites commonly charge a fixed price per click rather than use a bidding system. PPC display advertisements, also known as "banner ads", are shown on web sites or search engine results with related content. Dental implant PPC advertising can be expensive in certain markets – but worth it. When you track the

sources of your leads, you can easily determine is this is money well spent.

Many people desiring implant dentistry make their buying decisions by surfing for and viewing dental office websites. That alone is reason enough to create a website attractive to both the search engines and the viewers.

Nontraditional Media: Yellow Pages

Many experts predict the demise of the printed yellow pages. Certainly, the Internet is driving nails into its coffin every day. In many larger markets, the time for yellow pages has passed.

Nontraditional Media: Direct Mail

Direct mail is another highly effective way to bring implant patients into your practice. The best part of direct mail for implant cases is that it's the least visible marketing technique. Other dentists aren't likely to see your direct mail pieces and won't have the ability to mimic or copy you. In markets where petty professional jealousies supersede rational thought regarding the business of dentistry, it's comforting to know that marketing complaints to dental licensing authorities over direct mail rarely occur. It's essentially off the radar screen of your jealous peers.

Available today is something called **micro-niche direct mail**. It uses data mining techniques that allow mailing list segmentation. This process has become very sophisticated in the past five years, but until very recently was limited to only the largest corporations because of its high cost. The system is finally trickling down to where dental practices can have access to the same sensitive information as the biggest direct mailers (credit card companies, for example).

There are dozens of other nontraditional media out there, so be sure to evaluate their value carefully, and always proceed with caution. It's your hard-earned money being spent, after all!

With All Media

Before signing a contract with any media source, run tests first and sign contracts *after* evaluating a specific ad's response rate. Only commit to a contract after you see results and ROI. Doctors routinely ask, "What should I spend on marketing?" For practices that perform numerous higher profit implant cases and rely on external marketing for the majority of their new cases, 7 to 10 percent of gross income is typical. If the advertising message is correctly crafted and an effective case acceptance system is in place, the range of return on the implant marketing investment is from 4:1 to 10:1.

Conclusion

When you begin marketing externally, be prepared to receive some heat from a certain group of dentists in your area. They don't advertise and think poorly of dentists who do. They will call you unprofessional—and worse. They will put subtle and not-so-subtle pressure on you to remain a member of their flock. It's safer for them that way.

> *There is not much collective security in a flock of sheep on the way to the butcher.*
> — WINSTON CHURCHILL

It's vitally important that you resist their efforts, maintain your character and stay true to your dream. Dental implant excellence awaits you. Another excellent way you can promote your brand is to create awareness of your practice with positive public relations: read on.

CHAPTER 8

Positive Public Relations

THE THIRD COMPONENT OF YOUR MASTER MARKETING PLAN is public relations (PR). Public relations is an especially effective way to promote your dental implant services. The number of ways you can harness the power of PR is only limited by your imagination. In this chapter, you will learn seven positive public relations strategies.

PR Strategy #1: Direct-to-Consumer Seminars

This PR strategy is my favorite. Our office does six direct-to-consumer seminars each year at a local hotel. The one-hour seminars begin at 6:30 pm on Wednesdays and consist of 15 to 20 minutes of heavy hors d'oeuvres and a 45–minute implant lecture. We typically have 20 to 40 people attend. Approximately 10 of those people schedule examination visits that very evening, and 10 more schedule appointments at a later date.

Here is how I recommend conducting your direct-to-consumer seminars:

- Choose a small but nice motel, hotel, or other meeting room facility as near to your office as possible.
- At six weeks and then again two weeks before the seminar, do a direct mailing to homes within a three or four mile radius of your practice. If possible, select people with $80,000+ household incomes.

- Have interested people RSVP to a dedicated phone line in your office. Make sure to take names and contact information when people call.
- Arrive at the event site two hours early with your receptionist and clinical assistant. Be sure your computer-generated presentation and projector are working properly. Some people will arrive 30 minutes before the scheduled start time. Be ready to greet them at the door, check them in on your attendance list, and capture contact information for anyone who just shows up.
- From the scheduled start time, allow 15–20 minutes for people to eat the hors d'oeuvres as you mingle with the crowd. Choose foods such as pasta that are easy to chew and digest so no one feels embarrassed.
- Invite the group to sit in their chairs. Set the room with fewer chairs than you believe will be necessary. Have chairs ready to bring out at the last minute if needed. This will create a "Wow! There's more people than we expected" atmosphere rather than a sea of empty chairs.
- You can create and present your own PowerPoint implant presentation or use the ImplantVision software like I do. After welcoming the group, show the ImplantVision narrated video *"What Is a Dental Implant?"* and ask for questions. Next, show the *Consequences of Single Tooth Missing* narrated video and ask for questions. Then, show the *Consequences of All Teeth Missing* narrated video and ask for questions.
- Show before and after photos of your patients as you tell their stories and how their lives were benefited by implant dentistry. You can even have one or more of these patients at the lecture.
- Allow five to ten minutes for questions and answers at the end of your presentation. Keep the entire event to exactly one hour.
- At the end of your lecture, introduce your team members and invite the people to schedule an examination visit. Have your receptionist bring the schedule so appointments can be made on the spot. You should reserve time on the schedule the following week so people can be seen quickly.

- Stay in the room as long as necessary to answer individual questions.
- The next day, send a thank-you note to all attendees.

PR Strategy #2: Stay in the Public Eye

Stay in the public eye by attending and supporting public events. Examples are:
- staff a booth at hospital health fairs
- attend PTA meetings at your children's schools
- join the Chamber of Commerce and attend their meetings and events
- attend and do presentations at business and civic club meetings
- join networking associations and country clubs

PR Strategy #3: Serve Those Who Serve

When people give excellent service to any member of your team, give them one of your business cards with the following printed on the back: "I received excellent service from you today. Our dental office would love to return the favor and give you the same quality service."

PR Strategy #4: Be Polite to Everyone

Anyone can be a potential patient. Be polite to everyone you meet. This includes the FedEx, UPS, and dental supply people who come to your office. You never know who could be your next loyal patient!

PR Strategy #5: Use Press Releases

Send a press release to the local newspaper when you complete an implant training program. Here's an example:

> **FOR IMMEDIATE RELEASE**
>
> FOR FURTHER INFORMATION
> Call Dr. Susan Jones
> 555-555-5555
>
> Dr. Susan Jones, a dentist with a private practice in Los Angeles, recently completed the *Implant Dentistry Continuum*. Dr. Jones spent four weekends learning the most advanced dental implant techniques from Dr. Arun Garg, a world-renowned implant expert.
>
> "Our office is now able to do an even better job of replacing missing teeth and stabilizing lower dentures with dental implants," said Dr. Jones, who practices on Rodeo Drive in Beverly Hills. Her website is www.susanjonesdds.com.
>
> ###

PR Strategy #6: Lunch & Learn with Referring Doctors (for Specialty Practices)

Once a quarter, do "Lunch & Learn" programs for referring doctors. Try to hold the program in your office, but be willing to travel to their practices if necessary. It's important to involve the other office's entire team as they are the ones who provide the most referrals.

In your one-hour Lunch & Learn programs:

- Use a PowerPoint presentation full of before and after photos of your best implant cases. You can discuss the cases while they eat lunch. You can also use the videos and animations from ImplantVision.
- Bring a book of before and after photos of implant cases you've completed and tell an emotional story about how each patient's life improved. A copy of the book you created for your reception area works well.
- Leave the book with them so they can show it to their patients.
- Provide them with a referral card to give to their patients.

- Offer complimentary consultations for their team members or family members.
- Save 5 to 10 minutes at the end for questions.
- Be sure to follow up every month to see if the practice needs more information—and ask for feedback.
- Personally deliver seasonal gifts to your referring offices.
- Follow-up with all the leads you receive and be sure to thank the referring doctors and their teams.
- Go back to referring offices once a year and do other programs with before and after photos of patients from their office.

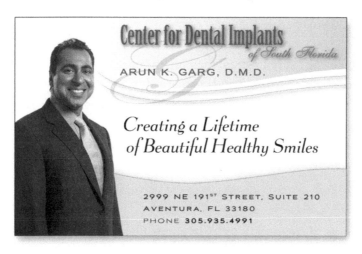

SAMPLE REFERRAL CARD, FRONT AND BACK

PR Strategy #7: Do a Local Smile Makeover

Doing a local smile makeover is a fantastic way to let your community know that you care about people (the emotional connection) and that you are an expert in restorative dentistry (the logical connection). It costs you nothing but some time and a lab bill, and can generate huge amounts of positive public relations with the people in your community and the patients in your practice.

First, establish a relationship with someone in a local media outlet. Local newspapers work best. They love the human interest stories of people in their communities. In many areas of the country, over 90 percent of people read their local papers. The next best options are lifestyle magazines or television/radio stations that do human interest stories.

Tell the media person that your office will donate your services to a deserving local resident who otherwise couldn't afford the procedure. Explain the steps outlined below. Be sure to stress the human interest aspect of the story: "This isn't a story about restorative and cosmetic dentistry. It's a story about a community member whose life will be changed for the better." Show the media person before and after photos of cases you've completed and the accompanying testimonial letters. Give the media person a short, written proposal based on the information below.

Timetable

The Smile Makeover is a series of events that follow the timetable below:

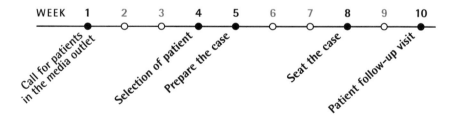

Call for Patients

It's best to schedule Week One in early September, January, February, or early March. In the media outlet, announce that, "Local dentist Dr. Tony Stark and the *Sun Times* are providing a Smile Makeover for a resident of Tallahassee, Florida. If you or someone you know has a smile that is negatively affecting their life, send a photo of the smile and a short story explaining why you or they should be selected to Dr. Tony Stark, 123 Main Street, Tallahassee, Florida. There will be no cost for the Smile Makeover. The deadline for submissions is September 28th."

Selection of Patient

Two days after the date you mentioned in the first story, review the cases you received and select the best three or four candidates. During the entire selection process, ask yourself:

1. What person will have a dramatic result? People who have missing upper front teeth or spaces between their upper front teeth are always good.

2. What person has a great story? Younger people whose social lives and work careers have been adversely affected are always good choices.

Have all the candidates come to your office and undergo a clinical exam. Be certain there are no significant perio, endo, or bite complications. The candidates should all have good oral hygiene. Sit down and talk with them for a few minutes. Ask a few follow-up questions concerning the story they wrote.

After you have seen all the candidates, make your selection. Notify the winner, have them complete a Media Release Form (supplied by the newspaper or radio station), and set a preparation appointment. Notify the remaining candidates who weren't selected with the following letter:

Dear Linda,

Thank you for sending us your photo and story. Even though you are very deserving, we have selected another person for the Smile Makeover. I hope you receive the dentistry you desire in the near future.

If we can help, please give us a call at 555-555-1234.

Sincerely,

Dr. Tony Stark

Preparation Visit

Schedule the preparation visit as soon as possible after you have selected the person. Have the person bring in photos from magazines of smiles she likes. Have the reporter at your office either during the entire visit or just at the end of the visit when the person sees their new temporaries for the first time. Take high-quality before and after photos. Be sure the reporter records the first words out of the patient's mouth.

If the reporter wasn't at the beginning of the appointment, review the smile design process you went through with the patient. Make sure the following four topics are prominently discussed so the reporter puts them in the story:

1. The patient works with you to co-create the smile of her dreams.

2. In response to your question, the patient tells the reporter how easy and painless the process was. "Peter, how did your visit go today?" "Any discomfort?"

3. The temporary restorations look great. "You can have a beautiful new smile in three hours at Dr. Smith's office."

4. The patient's emotional reaction is the primary thing you want to capture. "Peter, what do you think of your new smile?"

Seat Visit

Have the reporter back for the seat visit. Take photos after the case is seated. At this visit, briefly discuss modern cosmetic dentistry, the materials you use, and your advanced cosmetic and restorative training. Perhaps show the reporter other cases you've done correcting different problems. Be sure one of the cases demonstrates your implant expertise.

Follow-up Visit

Schedule the patient to see a professional photographer one week after the seat visit. At the follow-up visit, have the photos ready to show the reporter. Have the patient discuss how his new smile has improved his life. Ask the question, "Peter, how is your life different with your new smile?"

Briefly discuss with the reporter that Peter's reaction is typical of the people you see. Be sure to use "sound bites" the reporter will record:

- "Change your smile. Change your life."
- "Peter's new smile changes the way the world looks at him—and the way he looks at the world."
- "Cosmetic restorative dentistry isn't just for front teeth. Back teeth can be restored to their original strength and beauty." Show some before and after photos of cases you've done.

Media Piece and Reporter Relationship

The reporter will probably put all the above information into one newspaper article, one radio show, or one television segment. Offer to do some cosmetic dentistry for the reporter. Maybe this is only whitening. Take great care of the reporter. Send him/her a thank you note. Make the smile makeover a yearly event.

Conclusion

In the last three chapters, you've discovered a variety of tactics: intriguing internal marketing, extraordinary external marketing, and positive public relations. The purpose of all these strategies is to increase awareness of your office or move people to take the next step. This is why your phone number and website address should be available somewhere in all your marketing.

In the next chapter, you will discover how to create a website that is attractive for the responders of your marketing to view **and** is attractive to the search engines which people use to find implant dentists. The power of "and" strikes again!

CHAPTER 9

Wow Websites

I DON'T KNOW ABOUT YOU, but I rarely use the traditional, printed yellow pages book anymore. Especially when it comes to high-end products and services, I find almost everything and everybody on the Internet. For an ever-increasing number of people, **the Internet is the yellow pages of the 21st century.**

Double Their Pleasure: Be Attractive Times Two

The majority of consumers in need of comprehensive implant, cosmetic, or sedation dentistry are researching, locating, and selecting dental offices on the Internet. To be wildly effective at attracting these patients, your website must be attractive in two ways:

1. Your website must be attractive to selective search engines like Google and Yahoo, which sift through the information in the 400 million websites and the billions of web pages on the Internet. Search engines are giant electronic libraries that index a large portion of the information contained in these pages. This is an important point to remember. Search engines don't just index websites; they index individual pages within websites as well as website elements like photos, graphics, blogs, articles, and video.

2. Your website must be attractive in the eyes of viewers. It's vital that your website is a first-class example of your office brand.

Eight Tips to Build an Implant Website Attractive to Search Engines

Because of poor design, most dental implant websites attract qualified patients about as often as Paris Hilton finishes a crossword puzzle. I've researched website creation since I created my private practice site. Through this experience, I've discovered eight tips for creating websites that are irresistible to search engines.

Tip #1: Create attractive content.

Like Audrey, the carnivorous flower in *Little Shop of Horrors*, search engines are hungry for information contained in web pages. Here's an example of this constant craving in action. If your practice is in Chicago, and a woman enters "dental implants Chicago" into a search engine, the implant page on your website may be listed high on her computer screen. Now, the woman can click directly to that page.

Consequently, the more properly created pages about implants you have in your website, the greater your chances of getting one or more of them to appear on the top of the search engine results for implants. In addition, the organization of the information on each page will be critical to whether or not you get first-page results. Cramming too many topics on one page dilutes the focus of your information and confuses search engines. Be sure to give each area of your practice and each service you offer its own page. Each page should should be optimized to include important keywords and phrases relevant to the page's topic.

In addition, be sure your website is unique. Search engines are programmed to recognize duplicate blocks of text found on multiple websites. Your website information loses its appeal to search engines when it has "cookie-cutter" copy found on lots of other dental websites.

Tip #2: Add or chnage one or two pages every month.

Search engines and consumers are looking for fresh, original content. Creating or changing content will also give you more pages to optimize with key words and phrases that attract qualified visitors to your site.

Tip #3: Add blogs and video to your website.

The word "blog" hatched from the combination of the words "web" and "log." Blogs are online journals where words and photos can be added without the aid of your webmaster. The key is to make sure that entries are added every week. Blogs are extremely effective in building rapport with website visitors because they are written and presented in a more personal style than traditional website copy.

Search engines love video. Include video testimonials whenever possible.

Tip #4: Establish numerous inbound links.

Search engines are fantastic at locating information on the Internet. Unfortunately, they don't have the logic to determine the *quality* of that information. Links connecting two websites are one way search engines attempt to judge the quality of websites. When other credible websites have a link to your website, the search engines see that as a vote of confidence for your information. Therefore, the more incoming links you establish, the better.

Ask your colleagues in non-competing practices, other medical professionals, dental vendors, and alumni associations to link to your website. Ask for links on websites of charities and community organizations to which you contribute and on media websites (newspapers, radio stations, and TV stations) on which you purchase advertising.

Tip #5: Purchase sponsored links.

If you would enter the words "dental implants Chicago" into a search engine such as Google or Yahoo, the top two or three listings at the top of the first page and all of the listings on the right-hand side of the page were purchased. Every time a viewer clicks on a link, the website owner pays a $.10 to $100 fee to the search engine—hence the term "pay-per-click advertising." Pay per click can be a worthwhile investment. But you must accurately track the amount of production your pay per click advertising creates. Be sure all pay per click people are directed to a landing page that addresses their unique desires. Do not simply direct them to your home page.

Tip #6: Obtain listings on website directories.

Find relevant directory websites and have your site linked to theirs. These may be national "find a dentist near you" directories, or local directories indexing other services. Some links require an investment, but many are free. Join the free ones.

Tip #7: Link your yellow page listings.

Make sure your website is found in online yellow page listings, and link sites such as www.yellowbook.com to your website.

Tip #8: Write articles.

Almost all newspapers and radio and TV stations have online editions. Many of them accept well-written articles from you. You can also write articles for article directories such as ehow.com. squidoo.com and ezinearticles.com. Make sure you include a link from the articles to your website.

Form a Relationship with a Credible Web Marketing Partner

Most dentists and their teams don't have the time or expertise to effectively implement the eight tips listed above, so you will want to form a relationship with a credible web marketing company that is a master at search engine optimization (SEO). SEO is the art and science of creating sites which attract the patients you desire. There are many peculiarities to the creation of dental websites, so it's to your advantage to work with a company that has extensive experience in the dental profession.

Ten Tips to Build a Viewer-Attracting Implant Website

Your website must be attractive to the search engines **and** to the person who searched for and clicked on your site. Here are 10 tips to make sure that happens:

Tip #1: Be on brand.

Back in Chapter 4, you discovered the power of branding, and you learned how to create your one-sentence brand statement, which you wrote in your journal or notebook. Please look at that statement now. This is vitally important because the style and content of your website must be on brand.

If people come to your website and it doesn't match the external marketing, public relations, or patient referral that got them there, doubt will be created. Something just won't seem right. And people aren't going to take action on something as important as implants if there is a hint of doubt present.

Tip #2: Tell your brand story.

All great communicators are masterful storytellers. With words, images, and emotions, your website should tell the story of Brand You. Stories are magical. They engage people's minds and hearts and move them to action.

The grand story of your website should say, "Welcome. We know you have fears and desires. We're uniquely equipped to help you overcome your fears and meet your desires. We have the experience, clinical skills, and caring personalities that make us your number-one choice for implant dentistry. We consistently enhance people's lives. Contact us now to take the next step."

Within the grand story, you should have before and after photos and testimonials of patients who have personally experienced the grand story described above.

Tip #3: Differentiate your practice.

In addition to yours, how many other websites do you think the person will check out? I've never seen the statistics, but I assume the answer is three or four. To many people, a dental office is a dental office is a dental office. It's your job to demonstrate that's not true. It's your job to show and tell them how your office is different—how it is uniquely equipped to provide the best implant care in the area.

If you're the same as everyone else, you're a commodity. And the only way to consistently win the commodity game is to be the least expensive provider. You don't want to play that game, because no one wins.

Tip #4: Create a balanced blend of words and images.

We've all seen the websites that were 100 percent content, every page packed with information so valuable that the writer couldn't stand the thought of diluting the words with images. Conversely, we've seen websites that were gorgeous to behold, but didn't give the information we wanted. The power of **and** strikes again. Your website should be a balanced blend of written narrative **and** photos, videos, and graphics—like a child's picture book.

The copy should explain what you do and how you do it—and be written and edited by professionals experienced in web writing. Don't do it yourself or hire the high school English teacher who lives next door.

Any photos of your team, your office, or you should be taken by professionals. The same goes for the "after" photos of your patients. Having well-done video on your website is extremely effective and will differentiate you from the other doctors on the web. The video can be 20 seconds of you speaking directly to the viewer. Alternatively, video can be used to demonstrate the wide variety of applications for dental implants, like the ImplantVision video on my private practice website www.SouthFloridaDentalImplants.com or www.GargDMD.com.

Tip #5: Make it easy to navigate.

Just like a retail store, the longer a visitor stays and the more things they find on your website, the greater the likelihood they will pursue a transaction. Unfortunately, you have only a matter of seconds to get visitors to click deeper into your site. Effective navigation and high usability is essential to get visitors to remain at your site. Here's how:

- Put your navigation prompts in places visitors expect to find them. Making visitors hunt for them will kill your usability and click-through rate.

- Don't camouflage or bury your navigation simply to make your site look pretty. Usability is the primary objective for page layout.
- Descriptions need to clearly identify what's beneath. Visitors scan for target keywords. Navigation that is too cute can be confusing. For example, "Artistic Results" is not as effective as "Before and After Photos."
- Prioritize your navigation element. Make your most important links more visible. Funneling visitors to target destination pages will increase the number of leads your site generates.

Tip #6: Make it entertaining.

Julia Roberts makes $20 million per movie. I made $100,000 my last year after 18 years as a full professor at a major university. The cold, hard lesson to be learned: people would rather be entertained than educated. So, make your website intriguing and entertaining—because you have only two to three seconds to grab their attention. Use video and animation. Show a wide variety of before and after photos accompanying the stories of how your implant dentistry changed people's lives. Have photos of your team and you and a short paragraph about everyone's lives outside the dental office.

Most dentists target their websites toward other dentists (and away from potential patients) by being way too educational. Education is typically logical in nature. Entertainment is more emotional. This is why it's important to place a layer of emotion on most of the logical components of your website. People don't care how much you know (logical) until they know how much you care (emotional).

Tip #7: Make it interactive.

Case acceptance does not occur at one point in time. Rather, it is a series of relationship-building conversations that stretch through time. Your website communicates to the viewer. How can the viewer communicate to you in a simple and direct manner? By completing one of the following six forms they've found on your website:

- Ask the Doctor
- Refer a Friend
- Schedule a First Visit
- Schedule a Recare Visit
- Register for a Newsletter
- Respond to a Special Promotion

Tip #8: Have a privacy policy.

With good reason, people are concerned about providing you with their e-mail addresses. A written privacy policy will help allay their fears. Go to www.bbbonline.org/privacy/sample_privacy.asp for an example of a well-written privacy policy.

Tip #9: Let your raving fans help tell your story.

Utilizing quotes and testimonials from patients who are thrilled with your dentistry adds credibility to your message. It's important to have a testimonial page and to strategically place compelling, emotional quotes on relevant pages throughout the site—which ensures these "pearls" get read. Start giving your happy patients an opportunity to support and participate in your practice and you will be surprised at their willingness.

Tip #10: Make it easy to take the next step.

There are four types of people you will encounter when it comes to their interest in taking the next step:

1. **Impulsive**: These people buy quickly so have your phone number and email addresss on each page. Impulsive people are only 5% of the population, but most websites only cater to them. Big mistake!
2. **Want to Buy, But Not Ready Now**: Offer them a free/discount coupon to intice them to take action.

3. **Need More Relationship Building**: Offer them information.
4. **Not Interested**: They will leave without taking action no matter what you do.

Conclusion

Just as you need to choose professionals to undertake your search engine optimization, you must also select experts to design your professional website. Because the search engine optimization and design are interconnected, be certain the designers and optimization people work together.

You've now completed the first two steps to implant excellence. Step 1 was to Build a Solid Practice Foundation. Step 2 was to Be a Master Marketer. Step 3 is to Make It Easy for People. Speaking of making it easy for people to achieve excellence, all you have to do now is begin reading the next section. How hard is that?

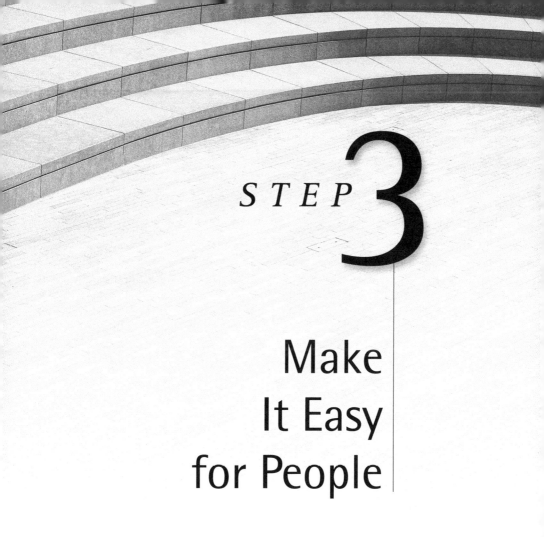

STEP 3

Make It Easy for People

YOUR FIRST STEP TO IMPLANT EXCELLENCE is to build a solid practice foundation with the four cornerstones of dreams, character, team, and branding. Your second step is to be a master marketer by marketing internally to your current patients, marketing externally to your community, and using public relations to shine a positive light on your practice.

Now you're ready for the third step: making it easy for people to say yes to the best care available—yours. Step 3 is incredibly important because I repeatedly see many dentists making three mistakes when it comes to helping people receive implant dentistry.

Mistake #1: Pushing people into accepting implant dentistry.

If patients feel pressured to accept care, they will take one of three actions: (1) They will push back in subtle and not-so-subtle ways. (2) They will protect themselves by erecting barriers that block communication. (3) They will leave your practice and not return. In addition, they will tell their family and friends about their negative experience with you.

Most people want the best modern implant dentistry has to offer. They don't always receive the best because of five barriers blocking their paths:

- lack of knowledge
- lack of trust
- fear
- inconvenience
- cost

So instead of being a salesperson who pushes people to accept care, be a consultant who makes it easy for them to accept care by removing or lowering each of the above barriers to implant case acceptance. I will show exactly how to do that in the following chapters.

Mistake #2: Assuming that case acceptance occurs only during the treatment conference.

Implant case acceptance does not occur at one single point in time. It's a series of small steps beginning *before* the first phone call to your office. In fact, **who's on the phone and what they've heard about you is typically the most important step to case acceptance.** If people hear that you're a fabulous implant dentist whose entire team provides excellent service, they will be predisposed to accept your implant care. That means you don't have to be a pushy salesperson; you simply need to be a consultant who serves people by orchestrating a coordinated series of steps that comfortably lead to most patients saying "Yes" to your treatment plans.

Mistake #3: Believing that only one person (usually themselves) is responsible for case acceptance.

Case acceptance is a series of events that involves *everyone* in your office. As a result, your team must understand the entire case-acceptance system in general and their specific place in the system. They will need training on how to effectively fill their roles in the system, as well as how to create smooth transitions to other team members.

Step 3 Preview

In the next three chapters, you will discover how to make it easy for patients to accept care by removing barriers to create a seamless case-acceptance system involving your entire team. Chapter 10 is your introduction to fantastic phone fundamentals. In Chapters 11 through 16, you will learn the art of creative case conversations. Finally, in Chapter 17, you will discover how to massage (not manage) money magnificently.

Imagine this scene: it's six months from today. Your marketing is pulling in calls from people who desire the kinds of implant dentistry you want to provide. How does each first conversation with every prospective new patient sound? That conversation on their first phone call is vitally important—it must be "on-brand" to lead to a patient visit. Read the next chapter to discover the fantastic phone fundamentals that will make this happen.

CHAPTER 10

Fantastic Phone Fundamentals

In Chapter 4, you learned about the power of branding and how to build your own, attractive brand. In the last section, you discovered how to create brand bridges to the minds of select groups of people with internal and external marketing, public relations, and websites. Now these targeted people are going to respond to your marketing efforts by calling you on the phone to schedule a visit. It's vital that the first phone call be on brand by exemplifying who you are, what you do, and how you do it.

This chapter will show you how to conduct these oh-so-important phone conversations. You will learn how to tap the power of your three tools of communication and how to be congruent. Then you will discover the ten things you must do during that first call. Finally, you will learn how to tailor the first phone conversation to each of the four types of callers you will be hearing from.

Three Tools of Communication: Words

You have three tools of communication at your disposal: words, voice qualities, and body language. It's vital that you learn how to effectively use each tool.

Patrick Henry knew the power of words. He stood and proclaimed, "I know not what course others may take, but as for me, give me liberty or give me death!" His words inspired a nation to declare its independence. Winston Churchill knew the power of words. During World War II, his call to Britons to make this their "finest hour" carried more power than any German weapon of war. Henry and Churchill chose their words very carefully. They knew that words are not just sounds: they are firecrackers that ignite *meaning* in the mind of the listener. And like a string of firecrackers, one lighting the next, the meaning directs the listener's *thinking* to a specific area... the thinking creates *emotion*... and the emotion leads to *action*.

Let's take a look at a series of word pairs that could be used in a dental setting and the typical meanings for each word. Which of the pair sends the on-brand message you want your patients to hear?

staff *vs.* **team**
waiting room *vs.* **reception area**
drill *vs.* **handpiece**
cut a tooth *vs.* **shape a tooth**
appointment *vs.* **visit**
interview *vs.* **initial conversation**
tell *vs.* **advise**
case presentation *vs.* **case conversation**
checkup *vs.* **continuing care visit**
cancellation *vs.* **change in the schedule**
pay *vs.* **invest**
discount *vs.* **savings**
bill *vs.* **statement**
pay for *vs.* **take care of**
contract *vs.* **agreement**
work *vs.* **care**
filling *vs.* **restoration**

You might be saying, "This is just semantics." You're exactly right—it *is* semantics. The definition of the word semantics is "the study of *meaning* in language." Meaning directs thinking, creates emotion, and produces action—three results not to be taken lightly.

In addition to the listener, there is another person who is shaped by language: the speaker. The words you choose to describe the people, things, and tasks in your office help define how you see yourself and your profession. Here are descriptions of two dentists. As you read these descriptions, ask yourself, "Which one would I rather be?"

Dentist A:
- meets with her *staff* in the *waiting room*
- *tells* people what *work* they need at the *case presentation*
- *cuts* teeth with a *drill* and puts in *fillings*.

Dentist B:
- meets with her *team* in the *reception area*
- *advises* people on possible *treatment* at the *case conversation*
- *shapes* teeth with a *handpiece* and places *restorations*.

> *A powerful agent is the right word.*
> *Whenever we come upon one of those*
> *intensely right words,*
> *the resulting effect is physical as well as spiritual,*
> *and electrically prompt.*
>
> MARK TWAIN

For the majority of family and restorative practices, a phone greeting such as, "Good afternoon; Morning View Dental; this is Holly. How may I help you?" is an excellent opening line. The greeting can be modified to fit your brand. I would encourage you not to be overly clever with your phone greeting. I've heard a few that were real head-scratchers.

Voice Qualities

Your words are *what* you say. Your voice qualities are *how* you say those words. Voice qualities include tonality, pitch, speed, degree of loudness, and variety. For optimal effectiveness, voice qualities need to be appropriate for the situation. In general, the person answering your office phone should be cheerful and friendly. She should also be skillful at matching the voice qualities of the caller. If the caller talks softly and slowly, your office person should do likewise.

The best way to evaluate your voice qualities over the phone is to record yourself. Then listen to the recording, notice areas that can be improved, and immediately do a re-recording which incorporates those enhancements. As a general rule, most people would benefit from increasing the emotion and variety in their voices about 20 percent.

Body Language

You might be thinking that this tool is in the wrong place. What does body language have to do with telephone skills when it's impossible to transmit something visual over the phone? Technically, you're correct. In the real world, however, a person's body language affects their voice qualities *and* the words they choose to say. That's why the members of your team who answer the phone should be sure to sit up straight and have a big smile on their faces while holding a telephone conversation. One trick used by many front office people is to have a mirror and/or happy face symbol in clear view.

Congruency of Communication

Not only do you need to use each tool of communication correctly, you also want to make sure all three tools—words, voice quality, and body language—are congruent. The word congruent means "in agreement." Have you ever heard someone use all the right words to tell you something would be done, but you still got a gut feeling that it wasn't going to happen? That's because the message conveyed by the person's voice qualities and body language didn't match his words.

Here are two sure-fire ways to be congruent when communicating:

1. **Come from a place of caring and service.** If you truly care about your patients and want to serve them, then your words, voice qualities, and body language will all match. Statements such as, "We're here to serve," and questions like, "How can we (I) help?" and "How can we serve you best?" are superb words to use.

2. **Have confidence in the entire team's clinical abilities.** Confidence or the lack of it is almost always manifested in a person's voice qualities and body language. That's why I'm such a huge believer in advanced

clinical training for the entire team. The education instills both the trainees and their co-workers with confidence that they can do their jobs well. And patients can pick up on this confidence a mile away.

Scripts

I think scripts are great. But for the scripts to have real power, the user must own the words. If you ask someone to use a script they don't believe in or that doesn't feel comfortable to them, you're shooting them (and yourself) in the foot. They either won't use the script because it's too painful to do so, or use the script (say the right words) but betray the message by the incongruency of their voice qualities and body language.

> *Words are the voice of the heart.*
> CONFUCIUS

So, when you want your team to use scripts, give them a sample script using the words you believe are best. Then have each person rewrite the script in his or her own words while retaining the full meaning of the script you provided. Then have your team members practice their scripts until the words naturally roll out of their mouths.

Ten First Phone Call Essentials

All ten of these should occur during the first phone conversation between your practice's representative and a potential patient.

1. **Answer the phone within the first three rings.** Have the person who is the best at getting callers in the door answer the phone. If she is busy, have the next best person answer the phone. If the phone isn't answered within the first three rings, have a message that says, "Thanks for calling. We're presently serving other patients. Please leave your name and phone number. We will call you back within 30 minutes." And then follow through on that promise.

2. **Write the caller's name the first time you hear it.** If necessary, have the callers repeat and/or spell their names. Mention the caller's first name two or three times on the call.

3. **Get them in the door.** Don't screen the calls by trying to analyze who will or won't be a "good" patient. We've all had patients whom we believed would accept comprehensive dentistry and didn't. Conversely, we've all had patients we didn't think would accept our comprehensive implant treatment plans who eagerly did, and paid with cash. Please resist the strong temptation to "weed out" the "bad" ones on the phone. Get people in the door so they can make the decision to accept your high quality implant dentistry treatment plans.

4. **Tell them you can give them their desires.** If they ask about anything within your scope of services, reply with, "I'm so glad you called us. That's one of the things we focus on in our office."

5. **Capture all their contact information.** In addition to capturing their first and last names, get their home, office, and cell numbers; mailing address; and e-mail address.

6. **Ask who you may thank for referring them.** If they answer, "My neighbor, Julie Garcia," ask them, "What did Julie say about us that prompted you to call?" If they say, "Julie had some implants done in your office," reply with, "That's right. She did. Are implants something a member of your family or you might be interested in, too?" If they answer, "Yes," they've taken one small step toward case acceptance.

7. **Establish commonality.** Discover something you have in common with the caller and talk about that for a short time. The commonality could be the referring person, familiarity with their area of town, someone you know at their workplace, or kids.

8. **Invite them to the practice.** Ask invitation questions that have two possible answers. Here are two examples:
   - "Your problem sounds like something doctor would want to check out right away. Does this Tuesday in the afternoon or Wednesday in the morning work best for you?"

- "We reserve time for new patients so you don't have to wait long to get in. Do you prefer something the end of this week or the beginning of next week?"

9. **Welcome them to the practice and ask a caring question.** After they have scheduled the visit, say the following, "Let me be the first to welcome you to our office. You're going to love Dr. Johnson and our entire team. Is there anything you would like to share with us that will help make your visit more comfortable?"

   About 80 percent of the time, they will answer, "I can't think of anything." This is fine. Just asking the question lets them know you care. About 15 percent of the time, they will mention that either they—or the person they're scheduling the visit for—have an extreme fear of dentistry, to which you answer, "I'm so glad you let us know about that. I'll let the whole team know about it, and we'll take extra special good care of you." About 5 percent of the time, they will give a variety of other answers.

10. **Preview the visit.** Briefly, let them know what is going to happen during the first visit. Then refer them to your website for directions to the office; health and dental history questionnaires they can download and complete; before and after photos of cases you've done that may be relevant to them; and/or pertinent educational material. End the call with, "We're looking forward to seeing you next Tuesday at 10 am."

*Every time you speak to people,
give them something to feel,
something to remember,
and something to do.*

JOHN MAXWELL

After the phone call described above, the patient's reaction should be, "Wow, this office is different. They didn't just ask me a bunch of insurance questions. They cared about me as a person. I'm looking forward to meeting them. I'm even going to call my sister to tell her how great they were."

Four Types of First-Time Callers

Not all first-time callers are interested in finding a new dental office as described above. Some callers are just interested in learning more about a specific service such as implants. Some callers are price shoppers, and others have emergency situations. Here's how I would communicate with each type of caller:

1. **Looking for a new dental office:** Follow the ten steps for communicating with people who want to find a new dental office. The bottom line: make it easy for them to walk in the door—and don't screen them.

2. **Interested in a specific service:** As your implant dentistry reputation grows, more people will call asking about implants. They may or may not be looking for a new general dentist. I would invite these people to your office for a complimentary 30-minute visit. No doctor time needs to be scheduled. When they come to the office, have a team member sit down with them in a private area and discuss their problems and desires. If appropriate, assure them your office can solve their problems and fulfill their desires. Show them before and after photos and testimonial letters of patients with similar problems. Give them a short tour of the office and introduce them to the team. Come back to the private meeting area and invite them into the practice by saying, "Joan, it looks like we could replace your missing teeth with implants. The first step will be to have you back for an examination. Would you like to schedule that today? We reserve time for new patients on Thursday afternoons and Monday mornings."

3. **Price shoppers:** Price shoppers can be an interesting challenge. Some experts say, "Don't even bother with them." I say, "If even 20 percent come to your office for a complimentary, no-doctor-time

visit, then it's worth talking with them." Many price shoppers are terrific candidates for the no-interest finance plans I will discuss in Chapter 13. Here's one way to talk with price shoppers on the phone.

Patient: How much are your implants?

You: That depends. What type of an implant are you looking for?

Patient: I don't know.

You: Okay, are you going to need any bone grafting with the implant to make it last longer?

Patient: I don't really know.

You: Hmmm, what quality implants are you looking for? Lower quality implants tend to cost less. Higher quality implants have a higher investment.

Patient: I never really thought about that.

You: Here's what I recommend we do. Let's have you in sometime this week for a complimentary visit. We can get to know each other better. We will show you some cases we've done that are similar to yours. Doctor will take a quick look in your mouth. Then we can give you a fairly good idea what your implant investment will be; and you can decide if you want to come back for an examination. In addition, we can give you some information on our no-interest finance programs. Does that sound okay?

Patient: Okay.

You: Great. Does Tuesday in the morning or Wednesday in the afternoon work better for you?

Patient: Tuesday morning.

You: Excellent. We'll see you then, at 9 am. In the meantime, check out our website, www.SouthFloridaDentalImplants.com.

Here's another way to handle price shoppers. When they ask you, "How much is a crown?" Reply with, "It costs nothing to find out." Then invite them in for a complimentary evaluation.

4. **Emergencies:** Some of your best implant cases come from emergencies. The callers may have avoided seeing dentists for years. With emergency calls, keep it simple and quick. Get all their contact information and schedule them as quickly as possible. When they come to the office, take great care of them: get them out of pain and schedule them for a new patient visit.

Time Period Between First Phone Call and the First Visit

The time period between the first phone call and the first visit is another in the series of events leading to case acceptance. In addition to referring them to your website, send them an on-brand, "welcome to our practice" folder. In addition, it's great if the doctor calls them a day or two before the first visit to welcome them to the practice. You can say, "Joan, this is Dr. Johnson. I understand you're coming in to see us tomorrow at 10. Katie mentioned that you (insert some personal information, the referring person's name, or a concern of theirs). I just want you to know we're looking forward to seeing you, and we'll take great care of you."

Conclusion

An old couple made their way down the mountain to see their first iron horse. As they approached the railway station, their hearts pounded faster and faster. When they saw the train parked at the station, both of them were amazed at its enormous size. Ma asked Pa, "What do you think?"

Pa replied, "I don't think it will ever get moving."

Just then the whistle blew and the train chugged slowly out of the station. As it progressed down the track, the train gained more and more speed until it was racing off in the distance. Then, suddenly, it disappeared around a sharp corner.

Ma asked Pa again, "What do you think?"

Still recovering from his shock, Pa replied, "I don't think it will ever get stopped."

Momentum is magical, with iron horses and with implant case acceptance. The train started slowly out of the station and picked up speed as it moved down the track. Implant case acceptance also begins slowly by people hearing about your practice from friends. Then they receive a direct mail piece from you. Next they see you mentioned in the newspaper. Now they have enough momentum to call you on the phone. They have a wonderful conversation with a member of your team. They're impressed with the person's level of caring and begin to feel understood. They visit your website and are blown away by the before and after photos. They receive a professionally produced "welcome to our office" folder in the mail, and a call from the doctor the day before their first visit.

They believe you're different from other dental offices they've experienced. They're looking forward to meeting your team and you in person. They approach your front door with curiosity and positive anticipation.

Congratulations! You've created case acceptance momentum. Now you must keep the momentum going by connecting with them during the first visit. Lucky you—and lucky them. Maintaining your momentum is the topic of the chapter you're about to read.

CHAPTER 11

Creative Case Conversation: Connection

D OES THE TITLE OF THIS CHAPTER sound strange to you? If it does, the strangeness is probably due to the words "case conversation." In dentistry, we typically use the words "case presentation," don't we? I believe there are important philosophical, psychological, and practical differences between the words "case presentation" and "case conversation."

- With case *presentations,* the information only flows one way—from you to them.
- **With case *conversations,* the information flows both ways.**
- With case *presentations,* the tone is formal. You're the professional telling the patients what you believe they should do.
- **With case *conversations,* the tone is informal. You're friends discussing what's best for the patients.**
- With case *presentations,* the process is rigid. You have a set case presentation agenda.
- **With case *conversations,* the process is flexible. You respond in unique ways to what patients say.**

- With case *presentations,* the patients reject or accept care in one big leap.
- With case *conversations,* **the patients make several small steps to the care they believe is best for them.**

Change Your Mindset First

In order to make the switch from the case presentation approach to the case conversation approach, you're going to have to make a switch in your mindset first. The case presentation mindset is, "I'm the expert. Here are your problems. Here is what I think you should do to correct those problems."

The case conversation mindset is, "I'm a friend and consultant who's here to understand you're unique problems, desires, and life situation. Considering the information you share with me combined with my knowledge and experience, here are the ways you can solve your problems and gain your desires."

I hope you're beginning to buy into the case conversation concept. I believe it's the right approach because it's more respectful to your patients. They will enjoy their time in your office more because they are active participants in the process. It's also more enjoyable and interesting for you. Instead of being a professional expert who commands, you are a consultant who understands and serves. The best part: this approach leads to higher levels of case acceptance. Now both the patients and your practice are winners.

Patient Care Coordinator

There are six stages of creative case conversation. I believe a patient care coordinator is the best person to help new patients move through these six stages. In some offices, the patient care coordinator (PCC) is one designated person. In other offices, the doctor's clinical assistants do the job. In a few offices, hygienists fill the role.

The PCC is the lead person in all interactions occurring before care begins. She:

- greets the new patients at the door.
- offers them something to eat and drink.
- sits down with them in a private room and gets to know them on a personal level.
- has a conversation with them to discover their concerns, fears, and desires.
- goes over their medical and dental history forms.
- takes them on a tour of the office, pointing out key features reinforcing the office as the one that can serve them best.
- introduces them to other members of the team.
- charts existing restorations during the doctor's exam.
- records the notes of the hygienist's and doctor's exams.
- assists or takes the patients' photos, radiographs, and impressions.

For simple cases in the $3,000 or less range, she:

- receives the doctor's treatment plans.
- prepares for the treatment conferences while patients are with the hygienist or are watching educational DVDs.
- presents the treatment options to the patients at the first visit.
- makes the financial arrangements.
- sets appointments for patients' clinical visits.
- follows up with patients who don't make decisions to proceed that day.

For more comprehensive cases, she:

- makes appointments for people to return for treatment conferences.
- prepares for the treatment conference after receiving the doctor's treatment plans.

- presents different treatment options to the patients at the treatment conference visit. The doctor may or may not be present. It's nice if the doctor sticks her head in the room and "blesses" the treatment plans.
- makes the financial arrangements.
- appoints the patients for their clinical visits.
- follows up with patients who don't make decisions to proceed that day.

As you can see, the PCC is the lead person in the entire new patient experience. PCCs have time to spend with patients and can say things about the doctor they could never say about themselves.

If patients don't accept comprehensive care, the PCC makes sure they come back to have *something* done. She keeps the completion of care moving along. Sometimes this takes weeks. Sometimes this takes months or years. It's vital that one or two people in your office are responsible for making sure patient care gets completed. If you don't have these people in place, a lot of patient care will fall through the cracks.

So who should you select to be your Patient Care Coordinator? The PCC should be someone who:

- **has natural communication talent.** Some team members are just naturally good at communication. The PCC wants people to have the best dentistry possible and isn't afraid to talk about that kind of care.
- **has a great personality.** She doesn't have to be a raving extrovert, but she should be empathetic and warm.
- **is enthusiastic about the care you provide.** It's best if she's been with you for at least six months and has seen numerous examples of your high quality care.
- **knows a fair amount about dentistry.** The best PCCs I know have been in dentistry for at least two years.
- **has the time to spend with patients and makes case acceptance her #1 priority.** This is particularly vital. In most offices, new patients get handed from person to person and important information falls through the cracks. In addition, the patients don't have time to bond with any one team member, and feel confused when yet another stranger appears.

- **is willing to learn a few simple communication skills** like the ones presented in this chapter.

Many offices need assistance when implementing the patient care coordinator position. Call us for our latest recommendations on consultants in this arena.

Six Stages of the Creative Case Conversation

Each creative case conversation progresses through six stages. In the following stages, I've used the word "you" to designate one or more of your team members, and the word "they" to designate the patients and the people who help them make their decisions. Each of these stages will be thoroughly explained in detail throughout the next several chapters, but to begin, here's an overview of how they all work progressively.

Stage One: Interest

> **You** offer an interesting service to them through marketing.
> **They** express their interest by responding to you.

Stage Two: Connection

> **You** connect with them.
> **They** connect with you.

Stage Three: Understanding

> **You** understand their life situation, unique concerns, and desires.
> **They** understand your office philosophy and what services you provide.

Stage Four: Education

> **You** and **they** become educated about their clinical condition through the examination and records process.
> **You** educate them concerning *possible* solutions.
> **They** educate you on priorities and which direction to proceed.

Stage Five: Solutions

> **You** provide *specific* solutions and make care affordable.
> **They** make the decision that's best for them.

Stage Six: Action

You follow up.
They follow through.

Creative Case Conversation Stage One: Interest

You offer an interesting service to them through marketing.
They express their interest by responding to you.

Stage One occurs before the first contact with your office. I've already discussed Stage One in the marketing section of this book. Creating interest is vitally important because who's on the phone and what they've heard about you can be the most important part of comprehensive case acceptance.

Creative Case Conversation Stage Two: Connection

You connect with them.
They connect with you.

Stage Two primarily occurs on the first phone call and during the first visit. Your success in life is partially determined by the choices you make. What isn't so commonly understood is **your success is primarily determined by other people's choices about you.** Do others want to work with you? Do they want to be your patients? Do they want to accept the best quality dental care from you? Do they refer their family and friends to you? If you have high levels of connection with people, the answer to the last four questions are, "Yes, yes, yes, and yes."

If you're only doing basic dentistry, you can have low levels of connection with patients and your relationships will be fine. If you want to do more comprehensive implant dentistry, you will need higher levels of connection.

> *Life is giving.*
> *Life is receiving.*
> *In short, life is being connected.*
> TIJN TOUBER

In the last chapter, you learned three easy ways to connect with people over the phone. You will want to keep the connection-creation going at the first office visit. You have three tools to work with: liking, trust and rapport.

Liking. It's a fact of life. People tend to do business with people they like. Think of the person who cuts or styles your hair. Do you like him/her? The answer is very probably, "Yes." The odds are very low that you don't like the person but are a customer anyway because he/she is a fantastic hair cutter or stylist. This seldom occurs because people rarely do business with people they don't like.

Here are six ways to increase the likeability quotient of your practice team.

1. **Hire likeable people.** We discussed this in Chapter 3.
2. **Give your patients compliments regularly** and encourage your team to do the same.
3. **Thank your patients for their loyalty** and encourage your team to do the same.
4. **Smile.** George Clooney and Julia Roberts have great smiles—one reason they earn over $20 million per movie.
5. **Use positive words and phrases** such as, "Absolutely," "Yes," "I'll take the responsibility to make sure that gets done," and "It would be my pleasure."
6. **Show interest in your patients' personal lives.** When you greet them, talk about personal things at first. Then do your dentistry. Afterwards, talk about personal things just before you part company.

Trust. Lack of trust is one of the primary barriers for people accepting implant dentistry. They must have high levels of trust in you as a clinician and a person. Here are four ways to be more trustworthy.

1. **Under-promise and over-deliver.** Trust is created when people's experiences exceed their expectations.
2. **Tell the truth.** This is an oldie, but a goodie. Don't shade or stretch the truth—it will come back to haunt you.

> *Look the other guy in the eye
> and tell the truth.*
>
> **JAMES CAGNEY**
> WHEN ASKED HIS SECRET FOR SUCCESS IN ACTING

3. **Don't be pushy.** Discover what they desire and then give them what they want in the way they want it. Be a friend and consultant, and treat them the way you would want to be treated.

4. **Relax. This could take a while.** Some people are slowly motivated to have comprehensive implant dentistry. It could be lack of knowledge, lack of trust, fear, inconvenience, and/or cost that are barriers to proceeding with care. Continue to talk to your patients about the benefits and continue to take great care of your patients until they are ready to say, "Yes," to comprehensive care.

Rapport. You create rapport with a feeling of commonality. The English language confirms this fact. When you have rapport with people, you're "on the same wavelength" or you're "in sync." Many dentists blow rapport by trying hard to be the all-knowing, all-seeing guru of all things. Their case acceptance philosophy is, "I'm the expert. Here are your problems. Here's what I think you should do." They consciously and unconsciously place themselves on a higher plane than their patients.

Get on the same wavelength with your patients by taking the following five actions.

1. **Discover things you have in common with people and have short conversations about the commonalities.** Use the information that a member of your team discovered on the first phone call. When in doubt, talk about the weather or some local news.

2. **Encourage your front office people to come out from behind the desk to greet people as they walk in the door.** This goes for you, too. Release yourself from the inner sanctum of the clinical area and wander out and talk to folks in the reception area. They will love it.

3. **Match their conversational style.** If you're speaking to introverted people who talk softly and slowly, match their style and talk softly and slowly with them. Their brains will unconsciously whisper, "Ah, a friend." The same goes for your extroverted patients who talk loudly and quickly and have a lot of hand gestures. Be extroverted with them. Their brains will unconsciously shout, "This person is on the ball!"

4. **Enter their world.** If you see people are struggling with justifying the investment in implant dentistry, enter their worlds by saying, "It looks like you're wondering if the investment in the implant dentistry is going to be worth it. Do you mind if I tell you what I hear from our other patients?" Or if they seemed perplexed with all their options in replacing missing teeth, enter their world by commenting, "You seem a little confused with all the options you have for replacing those teeth. Would you like me to clarify your options?"

5. **Use the connection responder.** Sometimes, we create mini-confrontations when we respond to our patients who make emotional comments. Here's an example. You quote a fee for $15,000 and the patient says, "Wow, $15,000! That's a lot of money!" *Don't* say, "I'm sorry you say that. We're proud of our fees. We use only the best laboratories and the finest materials to create the best restorations possible. Doctor has taken numerous, advanced dentistry training programs so she's an expert at doing the crowns and onlays you need."

    What does that reply do? It creates a mini-confrontation, doesn't it? The patient is saying, "That's a lot of money!" You're countering with, "No, it's not. If you knew everything involved, you wouldn't have that opinion." While your reply may be true in a logical sense, the comment disconnects you from the person in the moment. Instead, use the connection responder. When the patient says, "Wow, $15,000! That's a lot of money!" Respond with, "I **agree**. $15,000 is a lot of money. **And** when those implants hold your upper and lower dentures firmly in place, it will be worth it."

    Here's another example. A patient calls you on the phone and says, "I'm so afraid to come to a dentist. I haven't been in nine years, but I have a tooth that's broken and hurting." *Don't* reply, "There's no need to worry. Our office caters to cowards. Everything will be fine." Instead, use the connection responder and say, "I **understand** your situation completely. We have many patients who tell us that at first. **And** after they experience our level of care and caring, their fears vanish. I'm going to tell everyone in our office your situation, **and** we'll take extra-special great care of you when you visit us."

Here's a third example. A patient comes to the front desk and blurts out, "I'm really upset with you guys. You said this was going to happen, and it didn't!" *Don't* reply, "I'm sure it was just a misunderstanding." Do respond with, "I **appreciate** you bringing that up; **and** let's go sit down in the back and straighten this out right now."

In these three examples, the first responses definitely disconnected you from the patients. In fact, they created mini-confrontations. What did the connection responders do? Instead of separations, they created connective bridges that included the best verbal connection word on the planet—the word *and*. There are hundreds of situations at work and in your personal life where you can use the connection responder. Just remember its three parts: "I agree and…," "I understand and…," "I appreciate and…."

Chunk It Down

You may be thinking right now, "This section of the book has a truckload of information. I don't know if I can implement it all!" I understand completely, and here's what I recommend you do. Take three of what you consider the best ideas from each chapter and discuss them at a team meeting. Then implement one or more of them in your practice. That process will chunk the information down into bite-sized pieces that everyone can swallow.

Conclusion

Now that you've discovered these effective ways of connecting with patients, it's time to move to the next chapter and learn how to understand your patients. One definition of the word "love" is "deeply understanding and caring for a person." So understanding is the first part of love. I don't think we talk enough about love in dentistry. We talk a lot about clinical skills, practice management, and net profit. Love is almost a taboo topic. Why is that? *What if* the members of your team deeply understood and cared about each other? Wouldn't your office be a more pleasant place to work? And do you think your patients can pick up on the understanding and caring atmosphere in your office the minute they walk in the door? You bet they can.

What if your team and you made it a point to deeply understand and care about your patients? Would that make a difference in how you approached your day? Would your patients feel the love—and respond in kind? How would their love make you feel and what would that feeling propel you to do?

> *As a physician who has been deeply privileged to share the most profound moments of people's lives, including their final moments, let me tell you a secret. People facing death don't think about what degrees they have earned, what positions they have held or how much wealth they have accumulated. In the end, what really matters is who you loved and who loved you. The circle of love is everything.*
>
> **BERNADINE HEALY, M.D.**

In the next section, "Step 4: Keep Your Promises," you will discover the two ways to deeply care for your patients. In the next chapter, you will discover how to understand them.

CHAPTER 12

Creative Case Conversation: Understanding

Now that your patients and you are interested in and connected to each other, it's time to move to the third of the six stages of creative case conversations. This third stage primarily occurs during the first visit.

Stage Three: Understanding

You understand their life situations and unique concerns and desires.
They understand your office philosophy and the services you provide.

It's a basic law of human nature: if you want people to understand you, they must feel that you understand them first. Said another way, **understand before you seek to be understood.**

As dental professionals, your team needs to understand your patients' life situations. Accepting comprehensive implant treatment plans is a big deal for many people. They have mortgages to pay, kids to raise, and gas tanks to fill. The investment in implant dentistry must fit into their budgets. The more you understand their life situations, the better you can help them proceed with care immediately, or at a later date.

You also need to understand their concerns and desires. All of your patients walk in the front door with a unique story that encompasses their concerns and desires. The first part of their stories occurred in the *past*—the dental problems they've experienced, the care they've received, and the success levels of that care. The second part of their stories is occurring in the *present*. This is the condition of their mouths and their life situations right now. The third part of their stories addresses what they want for their *future* dental health and appearance.

The best way to understand people's stories is to listen, observe, and ask great questions. During the first visit, you will have several chances to pose these questions. The first opportunity is when a member of your team sits down with the patients (ideally in a private area) and holds the before-the-examination conversation.

Before-the-Examination Conversation

Use the information garnered during the first phone call to have a "small talk" conversation at the beginning of the patient's first visit. Then, preview the conversation to follow by saying, "Maria, we want to provide personalized care for all our patients. We want to learn your concerns and desires so we can help you have the dental health and appearance that you truly want. In order for us to give you that kind of care, I'd like to ask you a few questions and write down the answers. Would that be okay?" Record their answers on paper in a nice leather portfolio. Clipboards with broken corners aren't on brand for most practices.

Here are the important elements of the conversation.

1. "We like to get to know our patients. Tell me about your family." Listen and ask follow-up questions. Then ask, "**Tell me about your work.**" Listen and ask follow-up questions. Then ask, "**Tell me about what you do in your spare time.**" Listen and ask follow-up questions. Learn at least ten personal facts about each patient. Don't discuss anything dental-related for the first five minutes of your conversation.

2. "**In addition to (information you've learned so far), how can we help you today?**" Always start where they are, not where you think they should be. As an example, ask, "In addition to the broken filling on the upper right side that you mentioned on the phone call, how can we help you today?" If their answer involves an interest in a specific service such as implants, ask them, "Are you interested in

exploring the possibility of having implants? We can talk to doctor about that in a few minutes." If they answer, "Yes," they've taken one small step to case acceptance.

3. **"What kinds of dental treatment have you had in the past?"** If appropriate, follow-up with **"Why was that done?"** Here's an example. The patient says, "I had a root canal done on an upper back tooth about five years ago." You ask, "Why did you have the root canal done?" The patient answers, "I had a big metal filling on the tooth. It got decay underneath it, and the nerve got infected." You ask, "Do you have any other big metal fillings in your mouth now?" The patient replies, "I think I have a couple of them." You say, "I'll make sure doctor checks them out for you. We don't want that happening again. Is that okay?" If the patient answers, "Yes," he or she has taken one small step to case acceptance.

   Now ask, **"What other kinds of dental treatment have you had in the past?** They may answer, "I had a tooth removed on my upper right side three years ago." You reply, "Was the tooth replaced?" They answer, "No." You reply, "That can lead to problems. Would you like to explore some options for replacing the missing tooth?" If they reply, "Yes," they've taken a small step to having an implant.

4. **"Have you ever had a negative experience in a dental office?"** If they say, "Yes," you reply, "Tell me about that." After they explain the situation, you say, "Wow, that's too bad. We will do our best to make sure that doesn't happen here."

5. **"Have you ever had any gum problems or gum surgery?"** If they answer, "Yes," you reply, "Tell me about that. **Do your gums ever bleed when you brush your teeth?"** If they answer, "Yes," you reply. "Oh, that's too bad. I'll make sure Susan, our hygienist, knows about your condition. She can help you with that problem. Okay?" If they say, "Yes," they've taken a small step to accepting your perio therapy program.

6. **"Have you ever lost any teeth?"** If they answer, "Yes, in addition to the molar on the upper right side, I've lost all my back teeth on the

bottom," you reply, "**Have you replaced the missing teeth with anything?**" They answer, "Yes, I have a removable partial denture." You reply, "How's that working for you?" They answer, "It rocks all the time and doesn't fit like it used to." You say, "There are other options for replacing those teeth. Would you like to talk to doctor about them when she sees you?" If they say, "Yes," they've taken a small step to having implants.

7. Give patients a hand mirror and ask them, "**What improvements would you make in the appearance of your teeth if we could easily change anything?**" They may say, "I wish they were whiter and weren't so crowded. I have a new position at my bank, and my smile is really important now." You reply, "There are several ways that can be improved. Is that something you want doctor to take a look at?" If they say, "Yes," they've taken a small step towards having cosmetic dentistry.

    If you see metal restorations in their mouths ask, "**What do you think of the appearance of those metal fillings on your back teeth?**" If they answer, "Not the greatest," you reply, "Would you like to explore the possibility of having tooth-colored restorations done?" If they say, "Yes," a small step has been taken toward some tooth-colored restorations.

8. "**On a scale of one to 10, with 10 being extremely important, how important is it for you to keep all your teeth for a lifetime?**" If they answer, "It's very important—a 10!" you reply, "Good for you. We will keep that in mind when we discuss any dental care you need." If they answer, "Maybe a two or three," you ask, "Why so low?" They may respond, "Both my parents lost their teeth before 50, and I've lost eight teeth already. I don't have much hope for keeping mine." Of course, it's best to discover this information early rather than late, since now you have an education and possible referral process on your hands. If you discover this attitude late, you may waste everybody's time.

9. **"I'm curious. What do you look for in a dentist and his/her team?"** Discover what they want, assure them they will receive it and make sure they do. It's interesting that over 80 percent of the time patients comment on relationship issues such as friendliness, not clinical expertise. The vast majority of the time people don't care how much you know until they know how much you care.

10. **"Is there anything that would stand in your way of getting the proper dentistry you need?"** This is where money may come up. I hope it does because you want to begin talking about money early. I believe the whole patient-money challenge is such an important topic that I've devoted the entire Chapter 16 to it.

11. **"Do you have any time constraints for the completion of your dentistry?"** If they do have an upcoming special event such as a wedding, discover the date and show them how their dentistry can be completed, "If we start soon."

12. **"Do you have any questions for me?"** Briefly answer their questions and/or tell them when they will be answered.

Additional Distinctions

Here are some additional useful phrasings for further follow-up questions. Often, the most important parts of patients' stories are a couple of levels down and require a little digging to discover.

- "Anything else?" "What else?"
- "Tell me more about that."
- "Give me an example of…."
- "When does/did that happen?"
- "Where does/did that happen?"
- "Why does/did that happen?"
- "I'm curious. Why do you say that?"
- "Can you be more specific?"

- If you have previously discovered some information in an area that your next question also explores, just say, "In addition to… (the information)," and then ask the question.

Use the verbal and nonverbal feedback from the patients to guide you in the amount of time you take and the number of questions you ask. You also may have to suggest answers for patients who need ideas. Make sure to review their medical/dental history forms and at the end of the conversation ask pertinent follow-up questions.

Always be thinking, "What parts of their stories need to be remembered so I can refer back to those exact parts when we have our solutions conversation?" As an example, suppose your patient, Maria, told you a root canal was done on a lower back tooth five years ago. The tooth had a big metal filling which got decay underneath it, causing the nerve to become infected. It would be wise to refer to that fact when recommending indirect restorations on her remaining amalgams that are breaking down.

At your morning meetings, have the team member who did the before-the-examination conversation recap the stories of all the patients who are coming in that day for their treatment conferences. It's important that everyone knows these stories.

Now It's Their Turn to Understand You

Now that you understand them by learning their past, present, and future stories, it's time for them to understand your office philosophy, services provided, and procedures. Here's an example of what your Patient Care Coordinator (PCC) might say:

PCC: Maria, as you've probably noticed, our office is a little different. So far today, we've taken the time to get to know your history and your concerns and desires. Next, we're going to take some records and photographs for Dr. Johnson and Susan, our hygienist, to use when they see you. You will meet Dr. Johnson and he will do a complete examination of your mouth and discuss with you what he sees. Then you will see Susan, our wonderful hygienist. She will examine the health of your gums and the bone around your teeth and, perhaps, begin to clean your teeth.

Finally, you and I will come back to this room and discuss our next steps. We provide four types of dental care in our office. First, we care for your gums and the bone that supports your teeth. Second, we restore any teeth that are decayed, broken, cracked, or have old restorations that are failing. Third, we replace missing teeth with implants and other methods. Fourth, we do cosmetic dentistry to improve the appearance of your front and back teeth.

If you don't have a whole lot of care to do, I will present your options today. One option will always be the very best care that modern dentistry has to offer. There may be other good options, too. After I've done that, you can decide how you want to proceed. You can choose to do all of the care, some of it, or none of it. You're in complete control of how we proceed. Okay?

If you have a fair amount of care to do, we will have you come back for another visit with any other people in your life who will help you with your decision. We do this because doctor wants to take some time to study your records, get to know your case thoroughly and prepare the different treatment options. Again, it's up to you to decide how you proceed.

We also want to make the care affordable for you. You mentioned that finances could be a challenge for you. If you desire, we can get you pre-approved with our financing partner for a no-interest financial plan that will allow you to fit the investment into your budget. Would you like to start that process now?

Okay, let's go see Dr. Johnson. He's a great dentist and has a wonderful personality. You'll love him.

Conclusion

You've now learned the second and third stages of creative case conversation: connection and understanding. With low levels of connection and understanding, you'll do just fine providing drill, fill, and bill dentistry. But if you want to do more comprehensive dentistry, you must increase your levels of connection and understanding. Plus, it makes dentistry a whole lot more enjoyable when you've built that kind of relationship with patients. You're less of a mechanic who does the same basic dentistry over and over, and more of a consultant who consistently performs the challenging types of dentistry.

Incidentally, implementing the creative case conversation system in your practice is going to be a challenge. Congratulations! Challenges are life's way of letting you know you're making progress. Continue making progress right now by reading the next chapter on the fourth stage of creative case conversation: education.

CHAPTER 13

Creative Case Conversation: Education

MARGARET MILLAR SAID, "Most conversations are simply monologues delivered in the presence of witnesses." She was probably thinking of her dentist when she uttered those words. Most dentists talk to their patients 90 percent of the time and listen only 10 percent of the time. That's not a conversation. That's a monologue.

I think many dentists prefer monologues. It's safer and more predictable that way because it doesn't require any creativity in responding to the patients' questions and comments. But safety and predictability severely limit case acceptance because patients never feel connected, only separated. Patients don't feel understood, but instead suffer like a student who is being sternly instructed. As a result, they don't move ahead with as much comprehensive implant dentistry as they should. That's why I spent so much time on connection and understanding in the last two chapters. But patients *do* need to be educated—just not in the old style. You'll learn how to educate your patients without alienating your patients in this chapter.

Stage Four: Education

You and they are educated about their condition via the examination and records process.
You educate the patients concerning possible solutions.
They educate you on their priorities and which direction to proceed.

Records

Stage Four primarily occurs at the first visit. I recommend that the Patient Care Coordinator either take the records or be with the person who does so. The PCC can pick up valuable information about the patients' condition while the photos, radiographs, impressions, and other records are taken. She can use this information later in the treatment conversation. The PCC can also continue educating the patients and helping them make small steps to case acceptance during the records portion of the first visit using the information learned earlier. Here are two examples of what I mean.

- In the before-the-examination conversation portion of the last chapter, the PCC discovered that the patient had a root canal done because a molar had a big metal filling that got decay underneath it. When the PCC takes the radiographs, she can say, "Maria, we need to take these kinds of x-rays to check the health of the nerves underneath those five big metal fillings you have on your back teeth. Sometimes we can detect decay under the fillings. Sometimes the fillings block our view. I'll make sure to explain to you what we find."

- The PCC also discovered that the patient lost a tooth on her upper right side three years ago that wasn't replaced, and that she has a removable partial that's not fitting well. When the PCC takes photos of the patient's face, she can say, "Maria, I'm going to take photos of your face now. Sometimes when people lose a tooth and don't replace it, the cheek can collapse a little bit into the space where the tooth was. I want to see how you're doing. I'm also going to take some photos of the inside of your mouth. I want to see how much bone you've lost on your lower jaw. That bone loss is probably why your partial rocks all the time."

The Handoff to the Doctor

Proper handoffs are vital parts of the case acceptance process that are neglected in most practices. An effective handoff has three parts: (1) the introduction of the patient and the dental team member and the relaying of some personal information; (2) the conveyance of all pertinent information the dental team member needs to continue the conversation (as an added bonus, the patient gets to hear the information one more time); and (3) the transference of power.

Here's an example of what your Patient Care Coordinator (PCC) might say:

PCC: Maria, I'd like you to meet Dr. Johnson. Dr. Johnson, Maria was referred to us by her neighbor, Julie Garcia. Both Maria and you are big Miami Dolphins fans. Maria has several large, older metal fillings in her mouth. She got decay under one a few years ago and ended up with a root canal on the tooth. In addition, she doesn't like the appearance of the metal fillings in the back of her mouth.

Maria had a tooth removed on the upper right side three years ago which has not been replaced. She has lost all of her back teeth on the bottom. She has a removable partial that rocks all the time. Maria has told me she would like to explore the possibility of having implants done to replace her missing upper and lower teeth.

Maria wishes her front teeth were whiter and not so crowded. She has a new position at her bank and her smile is becoming more important now. She also has her daughter's wedding coming up in June. Maria says it's extremely important that she keeps all her remaining teeth.

Maria, you're in great hands with Dr. Johnson. He's a wonderful dentist and has taken lots of continuing education courses in implant and cosmetic dentistry.

The Examination Conversation

Did you notice that I placed the examination *under* the education stage of creative case conversation? I did this because a well-done examination is educational for your patients and you when you keep the information flowing in both directions.

So, before you don your mask, eyewear, and gloves and recline the patient, sit in front of her at eye-level and have a short conversation about your mutual friend, Julie, and some other areas of common interest. Only then do you recline the patient and begin your exam.

Don't talk in code as you do your exam and charting. Before you begin, tell the patient you're going to be using patient-friendly language. Conduct a thorough examination where you tell them what you see and voice your concerns for any problems. As an example, *don't* say, "Tooth #2 has a failing MODBL amalgam on it." Say, "Maria's upper right second molar has an extremely large metal filling on all five sides of the tooth. Wow, the filling must take up 90 percent of the tooth! I'm really concerned because my instrument is sticking when I feel the edges of the filling. I'm afraid the tooth has some decay under it just like the one where Maria ended up having a root canal done."

As you do your exam and charting, use emotional phrases such as, "I'm *concerned* about that huge metal filling on Maria's upper right first molar." "I *worried* about the bone loss I see in the areas where Maria has lost her teeth." "The bleeding around Maria's upper molars is the beginning of a *serious* problem." Many dentists are way too logical. Add a layer of emotion in most of your patient conversations.

In addition to being emotional and logical, use the show-and-ask technique when you see a problem. Here's an example, "Maria, take a look at the photo on the monitor. Do you see the area where you lost that top tooth? Do you see how the bone is melting away from the area as compared with the bone around the teeth that are still there? Take a look at this next photo. Do you see how the tooth in front of the space is beginning to lean backwards? I'm worried that with time you may lose the teeth around the space. That might have happened to your teeth in the back on both sides of your lower jaw. If you're interested, we can show you a great way to take care of these situations. Okay?"

Preferably, the PCC is in the room recording the doctor's findings and listening to his comments. At the end of the examination, the doctor tells the PCC which of three paths the conversation should follow:

1. **Comprehensive Care Path.** For patients like Maria who need comprehensive care, the patient and the PCC will have a generalized conversation about *possible* care to be completed at the end of the examination visit. Then the patient returns for a second consultation visit in one week so the doctor has time to study the case and create the comprehensive treatment plans.

2. **Routine Care Path.** For patients who only need routine care (two or three restorations, for example), the patient and the PCC will discuss the care to be completed at the end of the examination visit.

3. **Foundational Care Path.** For patients who have serious foundational problems (periodontal, endodontic, implant, and/or surgical) requiring care *before* you discuss a comprehensive restorative plan, the patient and the PCC will have a conversation about the specific foundational care to be completed. Many foundational care patients have not been to a dental office for years because of their extreme fear. They are often excellent candidates for sedation dentistry. Foundational care solutions costing less than $3,000 to $4,000 can be discussed at the first visit. Foundational care that costs more is usually best discussed at a second visit.

The Handoff to the Hygienist

Depending on your first visit protocol, it may be time for the patient to see the hygienist. Here's how the PCC should do the handoff: "Maria, this is our hygienist, Susan. Susan, Maria was referred to us by our good friend, Julie Garcia. Maria works at the Regions Bank on Ocean Boulevard. Maria says her teeth bleed when she brushes them and Dr. Johnson mentioned that the bleeding around her upper molars was becoming a serious problem. Maria told me that it's extremely important that she keeps all her remaining teeth. Maria, you're going to love Susan. She's a fantastic hygienist. I'll be back in 45 minutes."

If the PCC is presenting the treatment plans that day, she prepares them now and returns to receive the hygienist's report and recommended treatment plan. She then escorts Maria back to the private conversation area.

After-the-Examination Conversation for Comprehensive Care Patients

At the end of the examination, the doctor told the PCC which of the three paths the patient should follow. Routine care patients as well as patients requiring less expensive foundational care should have their solutions conversations at the end of the first visit. These patients will decide how they want to proceed, financial arrangements will be made, and clinical visits set. You will learn how to do all this in the next chapter.

The patients on the comprehensive care path will only discuss possibilities at the end of the first visit. These patients will return for a second visit for their solutions conversations where specific solutions will be discussed.

Because Maria is on the comprehensive care path, the PCC escorts her back to the private discussion area where they discuss the possibilities in the four types of dental care where Maria is having challenges: gum and bone dentistry, restorative dentistry, tooth replacement dentistry, and cosmetic dentistry. With comprehensive cases like Maria's, you're only discussing the possible care—nothing specific. In addition, you give Maria a rough idea of how much her investment will be for each type of care. With this information, Maria can tell the PCC how she would like to proceed. Please remember, Maria is not making final decisions on treatment in this office conversation.

Sample After-the-Examination Conversation

Here is how the after-the-examination conversation might go.

PCC: Maria, I know you received a lot of information today. What we're going to do now is sit back, relax, and talk in general terms about some of the possibilities you have for your dental care. We're not going to make any final decisions today. We will have you come back in a week with any person who will help you make your decision. Okay?

The first area we need to take a look at is your gums and the bone around your teeth. I know both Dr. Johnson and Susan were concerned about your bleeding gums and the loss of bone around your teeth. Take a look at these photos showing the infection around your teeth and these x-rays showing how the bone supporting your teeth is gradually melting away. You have three choices in treating your disease. Your first choice is, you can do nothing. This is not a good choice for someone like you who wants to keep her teeth. Your second choice is to continue having your teeth cleaned every six months like you have been. The problem with this choice is your disease will continue to progress like it has been. Your third choice is to complete Susan's three-visit, gum-and-bone therapy program. Together with the improved hygiene at home, which Susan discussed today, the gum and bone therapy program will get your infection problem under control. The fee for this program is usually around $900.

The second area we need to address is restoring those five back teeth with the large metal fillings on them. I know doctor was especially concerned about the molar on your upper right side having a crack in the filling. Here's a close-up photo of the tooth showing the crack. Take a look at the photos of the other four teeth with large metal fillings. Do you see how the edges of the fillings are crumbling? Those are the areas where doctor's instrument was sticking. We know those metal fillings are leaking and there may be decay under one or more of them.

Again, you have three choices with these teeth. Your first choice is to do nothing. The problem with this choice is that the fillings will continue to leak and the decay will eventually reach the nerves of the teeth. This is what happened on the upper left molar tooth where you had the root canal and crown done. Your second choice is to have the metal fillings removed and have new metal or tooth-colored fillings placed. The problem with that is the new fillings will be even larger than the ones you have now. They will last a few months or a few years, but they're not a long-term solution. We don't place metal fillings like that in our office.

We only do tooth-colored fillings when they are smaller and there is more supporting tooth structure. If you did have those fillings done in another office, the fee would probably be around $300 to $400 per tooth. Your third choice is to have laboratory constructed, tooth-colored onlays and crowns put on the five teeth. I have these restorations in my mouth. Here, take a look at this model showing how onlays and crowns fit on teeth. The great advantage to onlays and crowns is their strength. Do you see how they hold teeth together instead of weakening them? They also look great, don't they? You mentioned earlier that you didn't like the appearance of your metal fillings. Here are some before and after photos of cases we've done. People just love these types of restorations. These restorations are typically about $1,200 per tooth.

The third area of concern is the one missing tooth on top and the four missing teeth on the bottom that are replaced by the poorly fitting partial denture. On the upper, you have three choices. You can do nothing and allow the teeth around the space to continue drifting. You can have a fixed bridge done by having crowns done on the teeth on either side of the space and connecting them. Here's what the fixed bridge would look like. The problem with the fixed bridge is the bone around the missing tooth will continue to melt away. A fixed bridge would be about $3,600. Your best choice is to have an implant placed in the missing tooth area.

On the bottom, you also have three choices. You can keep using your poorly fitting partial denture; you can have a new partial denture made; or you can have implants placed. I'm going to show you some 3-D animations and narrated videos to explain the negative consequences of missing teeth and the treatment op-

---

[1] The best in-office tool I've discovered for adding an impressive, effective and efficient visual element to Office Conversation #3 is *Patient-VU* by ImplantVision. Whether your patients are missing a single tooth, several teeth, or all of their teeth, Patient-VU has a library of comprehensive 3-D animations and narrated videos your team can use to educate patients on the negative consequences of missing teeth and the implant treatment options available to

tions you have for replacing them. *(Show the appropriate parts of the* Patient-VU *DVD.[1])*

Do you have any questions about what you just saw? As you learned, implants are usually the best way to replace missing teeth. However, we could make you a new lower partial on the bottom for about $1,500. Each implant and the restoration placed on it is about $2,400 per tooth. You have one tooth to be replaced on the top and four on the bottom.

The fourth area you wanted us to look at was the discoloration and crowding of your front teeth. I know this is important to you because of your new position at the bank and the big wedding in June. You have three options here also. The first is to do nothing. With this option, the discoloration will gradually get worse. The crowding will very probably stay the same. The second option is to have your teeth whitened. Of course, this would make your teeth whiter, but it wouldn't improve the crowding. The fee for whitening in our office is between $500 and $800.

Your third option is to have veneers on the front teeth. This would make your teeth whiter and take care of the crowding. On this demonstration model, you can see what veneer looks like. Here are the before and after photos of cases we've done that are similar to yours. Our fee per veneer is $1,200 per tooth. We can talk with the doctor to see how many he would recommend for you.

Maria, I know that's a lot of information in a short period of time. I also know we're talking about a fair amount of money. I don't want to embarrass you. Maybe I shouldn't have mentioned the implants and veneers?

---

replace them. You can even use *Patient-VU* to produce take-home DVD's and full-color printed materials.

Patient-VU can be used with any Windows-based desktop, notebook, or tablet PC and is designed for use in the conversation room, treatment room, or reception area. I like the fact that ImplantVision guarantees you will save time and increase case acceptance within the first 30 days or the company will refund your investment. Go to www.implantvision.net for more information, or call them at 800-571-8812.

(Pause here. Maria will very probably make an affirming comment. If not, you need to deal with her concerns now.)

PCC: I just want to get a general idea of how you want to proceed. We're here to serve you. We can do the best dental care in the four areas all at once; we can do the care in stages; or we can do nothing right now. You're in complete control of how we proceed. Okay?

Concerning your gum and bone disease, do you want to explore the possibility of doing the periodontal therapy program?

Maria: Yes.

PCC: Great. How about looking at replacing the five big metal fillings with laboratory constructed onlays and crowns?

Maria: Yeah, I'll take a look at doing those.

PCC: Excellent. How about replacing the missing teeth with implants?

Maria: Boy, I don't know. Maybe replace the upper missing tooth now and do the lower implants later.

PCC: I understand completely. I'll include the upper implant in one of your plans. What are your thoughts on doing the whitening or veneers?

Maria: I'm afraid the veneers will have to wait. I may want the whitening if we can do it before June.

PCC: Between now and when you return next week, doctor will examine your case more completely and create two or three treatment plans based on how you want us to move forward. I will put together a couple of ways you can spread out the investment through time as we discussed earlier. Of course, we will get you your maximum insurance benefit.

Maria: That would be great.

PCC: Is there anyone who will be helping you make your decision? I ask because that person should come in with you next time to receive the same information as you and to ask any questions they may have.

Maria: My husband Maurice should probably come.

PCC: Great. Let's go schedule a time for you two. Here is a DVD of the implant information you saw today and some copies of the before and after photos I showed you.

Conversation Debrief

You may be thinking right now, "Wow, that's a lot of information in one short meeting. Maria will never remember all that." You're right. She won't remember all of it, but she will remember some of it. She will hear it again in a week when Maria and Maurice return for their solutions conversation. Think of the above discussion with Maria as an intermediate conversation. She hears about her clinical condition in four areas. She is briefly exposed to the treatment options and approximate costs. She doesn't have to make any final treatment or financial decisions. She only points you in the direction she would like proceed.

In fact, Maria gave her permission to talk about comprehensive dentistry. Remember when the PCC said, "I also know spending that much money may be completely out of the question for your family at this time. I certainly don't want to embarrass you. Maybe I shouldn't have mentioned the implants and veneers?" Think about it. What substitute can you think of for this after-the-examination conversation for your comprehensive patients? What alternatives are there?

- **Bad Option #1.** Don't give your patients treatment options and just discuss ideal care. Not only is this unethical, but it also can create doubt in people's minds. They may have thoughts like, "Why didn't he say anything about replacing the metal fillings with bigger metal fillings.? That's what's happened three or four times already. And why didn't he mention the possibility of having a new partial denture? It would be a lot less expensive that way. He sure was pushing those implants hard." You want to remove as much doubt from people's minds because **doubt can squash comprehensive case acceptance.**

- **Bad Option #2.** Give your patients all the clinical information, discuss treatment possibilities, dump a huge fee on them, present all your investment options and ask them to make their final decision—all in a 30-minute period of time! That's what most dental offices do, and then they wonder why their comprehensive case acceptance rate is so low.

Ending on a Note of Hope

With patients like Maria who have a lot of care to be completed, be sure to send them out the door with hope. Put your hand on her shoulder and say, "Maria, I know you have a lot of care to be done. Keep your chin up. Together, we will create a dental health plan that will get you back on track. Next week will be our first step. Okay?"

Now, schedule Maria's next visit right on the spot or walk her to the front desk to schedule it. Say, "Maria, you met Blanche earlier. Blanche, would you schedule Maria and her husband a visit with the doctor and me in a week? Maria has a couple of areas the doctor is concerned about. We need to get started with them soon."

Conclusion

Many dental offices approach education like most schools do: there's a special room with one person who is in charge of teaching, and the information only flows one way. I encourage you to be different. Allow education to happen everywhere in your office, at anytime, with anyone. Make sure that the information flows both ways so that everyone is simultaneously a teacher and a student. It's not as neat and tidy that way, but it's a heck of a lot more effective—and fun.

Now that your patients are interested, connected, understood, and educated, it's time to discuss the fifth stage of creative case conversation: solutions.

CHAPTER 14

Creative Case Conversation: Solutions

IT'S TIME FOR A BRIEF REVIEW of the creative case conversation process. The first stage is interest. You present your brand to the community with internal marketing, external marketing, and public relations. Some people are attracted to the words, images, and emotions of your brand and visit your website or give you a call. If the people who visit your website find it does a fantastic job of describing who you are, what you do, and how you do it, they will phone your office.

When you speak with them on the phone, stage two begins. You connect with them, and they connect with you. Soon, they walk in your door with high expectations. Those expectations are exceeded since the level of connection increases at their very first visit.

You move to stage three as you begin to understand their life situation and unique set of concerns and desires in the before-the-examination conversation. At the end of this exchange, they understand your office philosophy and the services you provide.

Education is the fourth stage of creative case conversation. The process kicks into high gear as you take records and conduct the examination. You talk in patient-friendly language as you show and ask. They *and* you become educated as you co-discover their problems in the periodontal, restorative, replacement, and cosmetic dentistry areas. You determine if they need comprehensive, routine, or foundational dentistry.

The education process continues for all patients on the comprehensive dentistry path and for the more complex foundational dentistry patients in the after-the-examination conversation. Here you discuss **in general terms** the care needed and the approximate investment required in each of the four areas. You use visual aids to show people why implants are typically the treatment of choice and how implant dentistry is completed. These patients indicate the direction they would like to take when they return for their solutions conversation in one week.

Stage Five: Solutions

You provide specific solutions and make care affordable.
They make the decision that's best for them.

The fifth stage of creative case conversation occurs at the first or second visit. This chapter will show you how to present solutions to patients on the routine, foundational and comprehensive care paths. In the next chapter, you will discover how to present solutions to patients on the comprehensive care path.

Solutions Conversation for Routine Care Path Patients

Let's assume your new patient, David, has three amalgams needing replacement. At the end of the examination, the PCC can have the following specific solutions conversation with him. Many dentists hold this conversation in the treatment room. I recommend having the conversation in a private area.

> *PCC:* David, you have three back teeth with large metal fillings that need to be replaced. I know the doctor was very concerned about the cracked filling on the molar of your upper left side. Take a look at the monitor. Do you see the big crack on the filling? Look at this next photo of your other two fillings. Do you see how the edges of the fillings are crumbling? Those are the areas where the doctor's instrument was sticking. We know these two metal fillings are leaking and there may be decay under one or both of them.

David, you have three choices with these teeth. Your first choice is to do nothing. The problem with that is the fillings will continue to leak and the decay will eventually reach the nerves of the teeth. I know this has happened to you before.

Your second choice is to have the metal fillings removed and have new metal or tooth-colored fillings placed. I'm sure you've had this done several times before. The problem with that is the new fillings will be even larger than the ones you have now—which will make them more likely to break or crack the tooth structure around them. Large metal or tooth-colored fillings are not a long-term solution for you. We don't even place metal fillings in our office. We only do tooth-colored fillings when they're smaller and have more tooth structure supporting them. If you do choose to have these fillings done in another office, the fee would probably be around $300 to $400 per tooth.

Your third choice is to have laboratory-constructed, tooth-colored restorations put on the three teeth. I have them in my mouth. Here, take a look at this model showing how onlays and crowns fit on teeth. The great things about the onlays and crowns are they are much stronger than fillings. Do you see how they hold teeth together instead of weakening them? They also look great, and you mentioned earlier that you weren't thrilled with the appearance of your metal fillings. Here are some before and after photos of cases we've done. People just love these types of restorations. Do you have any questions about them?

Your investment to do these three restorations is $3,600. It looks like your insurance will pay $800. That leaves $2,800. Take a look at this Dental Care Agreement. The restorations we just discussed are listed at the top. There are four ways to take care of the $2,800. Your first option is to pay in advance with cash or a check and receive a 5 percent accounting courtesy of $140. That leaves you a balance of $2,660. Your second option is to use a credit card and earn some frequent flyer miles. Your third option is to use the 18-month no-interest financial plan you've already qualified for. In that case, it would be about $150 a month. Your fourth option is the 36-month extended pay plan which does include finance charges. With this option, it would be around $105 a month. Which of the four options works best for you?

David: I guess the 18-month, no-interest plan.

PCC: Great, I'll circle that option on the agreement. Would please initial these three areas and okay the agreement at the bottom? Thanks.

Preferably, the PCC completes the paper work and schedules the restorative visits on the spot. If not, the financial coordinator comes into the room and receives the following handoff:

PCC: David, you met Blanche earlier. Blanche, David has decided to do three, tooth-colored restorations. His investment is $3,600. His insurance will pay about $800 leaving a balance of $2,800. David has decided to use the 18-month, no-interest plan. I told him his payments would be about $150. Would you please make the financial arrangements and schedule his two visits. Doctor is very concerned about one of the teeth so we need to get him back as soon as possible.

David, Blanche is a pro at making dental care affordable. She will take great care of you. We'll see you soon.

David's dental care agreement is on the next page. I recommend you modify the dental care agreement to fit your practice's unique situation, have it professionally designed, and then print it on a white paper version of your letterhead.

Dental Care Agreement

David Nelson   September 15, 2012

CARE COVERED BY THIS AGREEMENT
    Periodontal   none
    Restorative   **three laboratory-processed, tooth-colored restorations**
    Replacement   none
    Cosmetic   none
    Other   none

INVESTMENT ESTIMATE
    Estimated Care Fee $3,600
    Estimated Insurance $800
    Estimated Balance $2,800

INVESTMENT OPTIONS
1. 5% accounting courtesy - $140 courtesy, $2,660 balance
2. Visa, MasterCard, AmEx
3. No-Interest Plan - 18 months, $150 per month
4. Extended Pay Plan - 36 months, $105 per month

COMMENTS *(please initial each understanding)*

- I understand that changes in my treatment plan can occur. The actual fee may vary from the estimate above. _____

- I understand that my insurance coverage is estimated to be $ _____.   _____

- I understand that I, not my insurance company, am responsible for payment in full for all care. _____

DATE   RESPONSIBLE PARTY

DATE   DOCTOR OR REPRESENTATIVE

Four Points on the Routine Care Solutions Conversation

In the sample conversation you just read, I want you to pay special attention to the following four important points.

1. Did you notice the use of the phrase, "The problem with that is…" after I mentioned a less-than-ideal type of care? This phrase communicates your opinion of every option you give. Patients want choices, and they want your opinion. Now they are armed with information to make the decisions that are best for them.

2. It was mentioned that David would need to go to another office if he wanted to have amalgams done. Not only is this being honest and upfront, it will also *decrease* the number of people who go elsewhere for second opinions.

3. During the handoff from the PCC to the financial coordinator, the PCC says to her coworker, "Doctor is very concerned about one of the teeth so we need to get this patient back as soon as possible." The patient also hears the message and sense of urgency created, which increases the likelihood that the patient will schedule a return visit and actually come to that appointment.

4. A dental care agreement was used while explaining the care. Whenever you verbally explain care and financing options, **show** them the written information, too. Now the patient just initials the agreement and okays it at the bottom of the page.

Solutions Conversation for Foundational Care Path Patients

For patients who have serious foundational problems (periodontal, endodontic, implant, and/or surgical) that require care *before* you discuss comprehensive care at a later date, have the following conversation.

> *PCC:* Mike, as you know, we have some real challenges ahead of us. I know you haven't been to a dentist in 12 years. I hope your visit went well today and that your comfort level improved a little. As doctor mentioned, we do sedation dentistry in our office. I think that would be an excellent choice for you. Here's what I recommend. Tell me if you think I'm on the right track. I believe it would be best to have all your foundational dentistry done in one or two longer visits while you are sedated. That way you can have a thorough cleaning of your teeth, root canals on two teeth, and three extractions all done while you snooze. After that's done and everything is healed, you will be much more comfortable. While you're healing, you will see Maria again for three very simple gum treatments. Most importantly, you will take great care of your mouth at home. Then in a month or so, we can sit down and discuss the options you have in restoring your mouth. Does that sound like a good plan?
>
> *Mike:* Yes.
>
> *PCC:* Great. Your investment to do all of that is $4,200. It looks like your insurance will pay $400. That leaves $3,800. Take a look at this dental care agreement. There are four ways to take care of the $3,800. Your first option is to pay in advance with cash or a check and receive a 5 percent accounting courtesy of $190. That leaves you a balance of $3,610. Your second option is to pay with a credit card and earn some frequent flyer miles. Your third option is to use the 24-month no-interest financial plan you've already qualified for. In that case, your payments would be about $160 a month. Your fourth option is the 36-month extended pay plan, which does include finance charges. With this option, your pay-

ments would be around $140 a month. Which of the four options works best for you?

Mike: The 5 percent accounting courtesy.

PCC: Great, I'll circle that option of the agreement. Would you please initial these three areas and okay the agreement at the bottom? Thanks.

Three Points on the Foundational Care Solutions Conversation

Again, I'd like to draw your attention to three important areas of the sample conversation you just read.

1. Don't overwhelm your foundational care patients with too much information. Just make it easy for them to take the first step. Once they are out of pain, comfortable with you, and less fearful, they will be much more willing to consider comprehensive dentistry. If there is a lot of foundational care, you may want the patient to return so you can present the treatment plan.

2. Take a look at Mike's dental care agreement on the next page. It's designed to be very simple. In the solutions conversations, your patients receive a lot of information. Now is not the time to overwhelm them with fine print and paperwork. If they finance care, there will be more agreements for them to sign at the next visit. You will also want to have them sign informed consent forms. Some great ones for implant dentistry are available from ImplantVision.

3. Unless they request it, do not give patients a computer printout of each service, teeth to be restored, code numbers, and the specific costs for each service or tooth. This just confuses people and creates the "menu syndrome," where people pick and choose items from the menu.

Dental Care Agreement

Mike Vandalay   October 22, 2012

CARE COVERED BY THIS AGREEMENT
    Periodontal   **thorough cleaning**
    Restorative   none
    Replacement   none
    Cosmetic   none
    Other   **two root canals, three extractions, and oral sedation**

INVESTMENT ESTIMATE
    Estimated Care Fee $3,600
    Estimated Insurance $800
    Estimated Balance $2,800

INVESTMENT OPTIONS
1. 5% accounting courtesy - $140 courtesy, $2,660 balance
2. Visa, MasterCard, AmEx
3. No-Interest Plan - 18 months, $150 per month
4. Extended Pay Plan - 36 months, $105 per month

COMMENTS *(please initial each understanding)*

- I understand that changes in my treatment plan can occur. The actual fee may vary from the estimate above. _____

- I understand that my insurance coverage is estimated to be $_____. _____

- I understand that I, not my insurance company, am responsible for payment in full for all care. _____

DATE   RESPONSIBLE PARTY

DATE   DOCTOR OR REPRESENTATIVE

Solutions conversations for patients on the routine and foundational care paths tend to be fairly simple and are done at the first visit. Next, you will learn how to present solutions to patients on the comprehensive care path. This type of solutions conversation is more complex and is done at a second visit. So stand up, stretch your body and prepare to stretch your mind as well. The principles are the same: it's the application that's more challenging.

It's time to rejoin Maria and her husband, Maurice, as they take part in the solutions conversation for patients on the comprehensive care path.

Solutions Conversation for Patients on the Comprehensive Care Path

With patients on the comprehensive care path, you have already discussed care in general terms during the after-the-examination conversation at the first visit, just like you saw with Maria. In that conversation, Maria indicated which types of care she wants to discuss at the next visit—and which types of care she wants to consider at a later date.

Maria and her husband Maurice have returned for a second visit where they will discuss care at the solutions conversation with the PCC and/or doctor. The conversation is similar to the first conversation with Maria, but is more specific now. After some talk about personal topics, here's how the conversation might go.

> *PCC:* Maria, thanks for bringing Maurice with you. My role today is to explain your options when it comes to the four areas we discussed a week ago. In addition, we want to make the care affordable so that it fits into your budget. We will make sure you receive your maximum insurance benefit, and we also have several ways you can spread your investment out through time if you desire. Your role is to decide what you want to do. You can choose to do everything we discuss right away. You can choose to do everything we discuss in phases—or you can choose to do nothing. You're in complete control of the direction we go. Okay?

Maria, there's a lot that is right with your mouth. The bone support around your teeth is pretty good. Your gums can become very healthy with just some care here in the office and at home. Except for those five teeth with the big metal fillings, your tooth structure is solid. Most importantly, I can see that you want to make your mouth as healthy as it can be.

At your last visit you mentioned that keeping all your teeth for a lifetime was extremely important to you. I believe you said it was a 10 on a scale of one to 10. You also told me that the appearance of your front and back teeth is important to you, too. Everything we discuss today is designed to help you achieve those two goals.

There are four areas of concern in Maria's mouth. The first area is Maria's gums and the bone around her teeth. At Maria's last visit, both Dr. Johnson and our hygienist, Susan, were concerned about Maria's bleeding gums and loss of bone around the teeth. Here are some photos showing the infection around her teeth and x-rays showing how the bone supporting her teeth is gradually melting away. You have three choices in treating this gum and bone disease. The first choice is to do nothing. The problem with that is the disease will continue to progress. Your second choice is for Maria to continue having her teeth cleaned every six months like she has been. The problem with that is, her disease will continue to progress like it has been. Your third choice is to complete Susan's three-visit gum and bone therapy program. Together with the improved hygiene at home, which Susan discussed last week, the gum and bone therapy program will get your disease under control. Maria mentioned last time that both her parents lost their teeth before the age of 50, and that she really wants to keep all her teeth. The therapy program is the best way she can make this happen. This program is $900.

The second area we need to address is restoring those five back teeth with the large metal fillings in them. I know doctor was very concerned about the molar on Maria's upper right side that has a cracked filling. Take a look on the monitor at a photo of that tooth. The other four fillings are breaking down. On these photos, do you see how the edges of the fillings are crumbling? Those are the areas where doctor's instrument was sticking. We suspect those metal fillings are leaking, and there may be decay under one or more of them.

Again, you have three choices with these five teeth. Your first choice is to do nothing. The problem with that is, the fillings may continue to leak and the decay may eventually reach the nerve of the tooth. This is what happened on Maria's upper left molar tooth where she had the root canal and crown done. Your second choice is to have the metal fillings removed and have new metal or tooth-colored fillings placed. The problem with that is the new fillings will be even larger than the ones Maria has now. They will last a few months or a few years, but they're not a long-term solution. We don't do metal fillings like that in our office. We only do tooth-colored fillings when they are smaller and there is more supporting tooth structure. If you did have those fillings done in another office, the fee would probably be around $300 to $400 per tooth.

Your third choice is to have laboratory-constructed, tooth-colored restorations put on the five teeth. These are what I have in my mouth. Here, take a look at this model showing how onlays and crowns fit on teeth. The great things about the onlays and crowns are they are much stronger than fillings. Do you see how they hold teeth together instead of weakening them? They also look great, and Maria mentioned last week that she didn't like the appearance of her metal fillings. Here are some before and after photos of cases we've done with the onlays and crowns. People just love these types of restorations. Our fee for these restorations is $1,200 per tooth.

The third area of concern is Maria's missing teeth. She has one missing on top that has not been replaced and four missing on the bottom, which have been replaced by a partial denture that is not fitting well. I'm going to show you some 3-D animations and narrated videos to explain the negative consequences of missing teeth and the treatment options you have for replacing them. I showed this to Maria last week, and I want to make sure Maurice sees it too.

Do you two have any questions about the video? You have three choices about replacing these teeth. Your first choice is to do nothing. The problem with that is the bone in the area of the missing teeth will continue to melt away. Take a look at these x-rays to see what I mean. This loss of bone support is why Maria's lower partial is rocking and why her face is sinking in a little bit in the areas where the bone is being lost. Look at these photos of Maria to see what I mean. Here are some plaster models of Maria's teeth. You can see how the bone has been lost in the areas of the missing teeth. Look on the upper right side. Do you see how the teeth on both sides of the space are leaning into the space? This tilting puts harmful stress on the teeth when Maria bites together. With time, many people lose the teeth around the one missing tooth. This may have happened on Maria's lower jaw.

Your second choice is to have a new partial denture for the lower. The problem with that is the bone will continue to melt away, and Maria will continue to have the hassle of wearing a partial. The fee for a new partial is $1,600. Your third choice is to have the teeth replaced with implants. As you learned on the video, this is your best choice. At the last visit, Maria mentioned that she would like to explore the possibility of having the top tooth replaced with an implant and wait to have implants on the lower. Each implant and the restoration that is placed on it is $2,400.

The fourth area you wanted us to look at was the discoloration and crowding of Maria's front teeth. I know this is important to her because of her new position at the bank and the big wedding in June. You have three options here also. The first is to do nothing. With this option, the discoloration will gradually get worse. The crowding will very probably stay about the same. The second option is to have Maria's teeth whitened. This would make her teeth whiter, but it wouldn't improve the crowding. Here are some before and after photos of whitening cases we've done. The fee for whitening in our office is $695. This includes a laser whitening procedure in the office and customized whitening trays and whitening gel for Maria to use at home. If we can start soon, Maria can have her teeth nice and white by your daughter's wedding day. Your third option is to have veneers on the front teeth. This would make Maria's teeth whiter and give her a beautiful smile. At our last visit, Maria told me she would consider having the whitening done, but wanted to wait on the veneers.

Do you have any questions about what we've discussed so far? Good. I know that's a lot of information, and I want to help you make the decision that's best for you by offering three plans of action. Follow along with these dental care agreements *(see Maria's good, better, and best agreements on pages 170, 171, and 172)* as I review three possible plans of action we've created for you. A *good* plan is to complete the gum and bone therapy program with Susan; have the two worst metal fillings replaced with tooth-colored restorations; and have the whitening completed. Your investment for the good plan is $3,995. We estimate that your insurance will pay about $800. That leaves a balance of $3,195 or about $269 a month with our 12-month, no-interest financial option.

A *better* plan is to do the therapy program; all five of the onlays and crowns; the upper implant; and the whitening. Your investment is $9,995 for the better plan. With the $800 insurance benefit, that leaves a balance of $9,185 or about $386 a month with our 24-month, no-interest financial option. The *best* plan is the therapy program; all five restorations; the upper implant; the lower partial; and the whitening. Your investment is $11,595. With your $800 insurance benefit, that leaves a balance of $10,795 or about $453 a month with our 24-month, no-interest financial option. We also have other financial options for longer time periods that would lower your monthly payments. Do you have any questions?

Excellent, we're here to serve you. Which of the three plans works best for you?

If another person is doing the financial arrangements, do the following handoff:

PCC: Maria and Maurice, you both know Blanche. Blanche, Maria and Maurice have decided to do this plan. Would you please make the financial arrangements and schedule Maria's visits? Doctor is very concerned about one of the teeth so we need to get Maria back as soon as possible. Blanche is a pro at making dental care affordable. She will take great care of you. We'll see you soon.

If Maria and Maurice choose the better plan, the person doing the financial arrangements says the following:

PCC: Congratulations on your decision. Now let's discuss your financial options as you follow along with the dental care agreement you selected. Your first option is to pay for the entire plan five days before Maria's next visit with cash or check. When you do that, you earn a 5 percent accounting reduction of $459. That leaves a balance of $8,726. Your second option is to use a credit card and earn some frequent flyer miles. Your third option is our 24-month, no-interest plan with a payment of $386 a month. Your fourth option is the 48-month extended pay plan with interest. Your payment would be $275 a month. Which of these investment options works best for you?

Maria: The 24-month, no-interest option.

PCC: Great, I'll circle that option on the form. Would you please initial these three areas and okay the agreement at the bottom?

Here are Maria's good, better, and best agreements.

Dental Care Agreement   GOOD

Maria Ortiz   December 3, 2013

CARE COVERED BY THIS AGREEMENT

Periodontal	**gum and bone therapy program**
Restorative	**two laboratory-processed, tooth-colored restorations**
Replacement	none
Cosmetic	**whitening**
Other	none

INVESTMENT ESTIMATE

Estimated Care Fee	$3,995
Estimated Insurance	$800
Estimated Balance	$3,195

INVESTMENT OPTIONS

1. 5% accounting courtesy - $160 courtesy, $3,035 balance
2. Visa, MasterCard, AmEx
3. No-Interest Plan - 12 months, $269 per month
4. Extended Pay Plan - 36 months, $320 per month

COMMENTS *(please initial each understanding)*

- I understand that changes in my treatment plan can occur. The actual fee may vary from the estimate above. _____
- I understand that my insurance coverage is estimated to be $ _____. _____
- I understand that I, not my insurance company, am responsible for payment in full for all care. _____

___
DATE   RESPONSIBLE PARTY

___
DATE   DOCTOR OR REPRESENTATIVE

Dental Care Agreement   **BETTER**

Maria Ortiz   December 3, 2013

CARE COVERED BY THIS AGREEMENT

Periodontal	**gum and bone therapy program**
Restorative	**five laboratory-processed, tooth-colored restorations**
Replacement	**one implant and restoration**
Cosmetic	**whitening**
Other	none

INVESTMENT ESTIMATE

Estimated Care Fee	$9,995
Estimated Insurance	$800
Estimated Balance	$9,195

INVESTMENT OPTIONS

1. 5% accounting courtesy - $459 courtesy, $8,726 balance
2. Visa, MasterCard, AmEx
3. No-Interest Plan - 24 months, $386 per month
4. Extended Pay Plan - 48 months, $282 per month

COMMENTS *(please initial each understanding)*

- I understand that changes in my treatment plan can occur. The actual fee may vary from the estimate above. _____
- I understand that my insurance coverage is estimated to be $ _____.   _____
- I understand that I, not my insurance company, am responsible for payment in full for all care. _____

_____
DATE   RESPONSIBLE PARTY

_____
DATE   DOCTOR OR REPRESENTATIVE

Dental Care Agreement   BEST

Maria Ortiz   December 3, 2013

CARE COVERED BY THIS AGREEMENT

Periodontal	**gum and bone therapy program**
Restorative	**five laboratory-processed, tooth-colored restorations**
Replacement	**one implant and restoration, lower partial denture**
Cosmetic	**whitening**
Other	none

INVESTMENT ESTIMATE

Estimated Care Fee	$11,595
Estimated Insurance	$800
Estimated Balance	$10,795

INVESTMENT OPTIONS

1. 5% accounting courtesy - $539 courtesy, $10,256 balance
2. Visa, MasterCard, AmEx
3. No-Interest Plan - 24 months, $453 per month
4. Extended Pay Plan - 48 months, $311 per month

COMMENTS *(please initial each understanding)*

- I understand that changes in my treatment plan can occur. The actual fee may vary from the estimate above. _____

- I understand that my insurance coverage is estimated to be $ _____. _____

- I understand that I, not my insurance company, am responsible for payment in full for all care. _____

_____
DATE   RESPONSIBLE PARTY

_____
DATE   DOCTOR OR REPRESENTATIVE

Five Steps of a Solutions Conversation for Comprehensive Care Path Patients

Every successful solutions conversation for patients on the comprehensive care path, including the sample you just read, consists of five steps. When you review the conversation above, you will see them all in action.

Step One: Set the Stage

Welcome patients back for their return visit and let them know you're excited to present their comprehensive plans. Hold your treatment conferences in a quiet and professional-looking room, ensuring you won't be interrupted.

Let the patients know what's *right* about their mouths.

Sit at a 90-degree angle to the patients so you can look them in the eye while easily showing them visuals.

Preview what will be covered in today's visit and clarify their and your roles.

Step Two: Rekindle Desires

Use the information you discovered in the before-the-examination conversation to create a short statement of the patient's functional and cosmetic desires. This will help you turn the conversation from, "I'm the expert. Here are your problems. Here's what I think you should do." to "Here's what you've told me that you want for the health of your mouth and smile. We're here to serve you. Here are three ways you can receive what you told us you want."

Step Three: Present Solutions

For each of the appropriate four types of care (periodontal, restorative, replacement, and cosmetic), give the patient two to four possible solutions. The first solution is typically, "Do nothing." With the "Do nothing" option, link the pain they may or will experience if they take that course of action. For the possible solutions leading up to the best solution, use the phrase, "The problem with that is…" When you discuss the best solution, show and tell them all the pleasure they will receive. After each possible solution, give them an idea of what their investment will be.

Step Four: Agree on the Good, Better, or Best Plan

Before the solutions conversation, prepare three treatment plans: good, better, and best. Use a single dental care agreement for each plan. I recommend the first one you prepare is the *best* plan. Remember that your patient may have indicated some care he or she doesn't want to consider right now—be sure to demonstrate that you've listened to their desires by *not* including those items. As an example, Maria didn't want to consider veneers and lower implants. Then create a *good* plan. This one typically includes basic dentistry and, perhaps, lower investment cosmetic care such as whitening. Finally, create the *better* plan, which falls somewhere in between good and best.

At the day of the visit, present the *good* solution first with the aid of a dental care agreement. Present the fee for that option. Then present the *better* solution with the aid of a second dental care agreement. Present the fee for that solution. Then present the *best* solution with the aid of a third dental care agreement. Present the fee for that solution. Then ask, "We're here to serve you. Which of the three plans works best for you?"

Step Five: Agree on an Investment Option

Using the dental care agreement for the plan they selected, present the four investment options and ask, "Which option works best for you?" Then circle the option they selected and have them okay the agreement.

Nine Points on the Comprehensive Care Solutions Conversation

The sample conversation is just that—an example for you to tailor to your own patients. Each conversation will need to be uniquely adapted to each of your patients. The following nine points will help you and your team do just that, and soon the process will be second nature to everyone.

1. **Blend their stories into your stories.** Take information from the past, present, and future stories you've discovered in previous conversations and blend those details into your solutions conversations. This will personalize your solutions and show patients how to avoid their

unique pains and gain their unique desires. In Maria's case, the information in her story included:

- her desire to explore the possibility of having implants
- her previous root canal and crown on an upper left molar that had a large, broken-down amalgam
- her parents losing their teeth before the age of 50—and her desire to not let that happen to her
- her dislike of her partial and the probability that her lower back teeth were lost as a chain reaction that began by losing one tooth on each side
- her desire to have more attractive teeth for her new job and family wedding
- her aversion to the appearance of the metal fillings on her back teeth

2. **Use the take-away principle.** At her first visit, Maria mentioned that she wanted to wait on her veneers and lower implants. At the second visit, the veneers and lower implants were mentioned in passing, but not included in the plans. Not only is that the respectful thing to do, but removing them from consideration makes having them more desirable. Her husband may say, "Maria, I would really like you to have those veneers, and your mom has mentioned she would pay for them. Why don't we think about doing them?"

3. **Use PowerPoint.** Using a PowerPoint software program is an excellent way to move through the five steps. It takes a little while to prepare, but it keeps you on track, and keeps the patients involved visually. You can also make a CD of the PowerPoint presentation and/or print it for your patients to take home.

4. **Cure the single-tooth syndrome.** This chronic disease is characterized by the symptom of patients only wanting to restore one tooth a year. It is sometimes called "the Crown a Year Club." There are two primary causes of the single-tooth syndrome:

a. The insurance cause: patients focusing on yearly insurance maximum benefits.
b. The iatrogenic cause: patients focusing on individual teeth because dental teams talk individual teeth.

In most dental offices, the creation of the single-tooth syndrome begins before the examination. The patient says, "I have a broken metal filling on the upper right side." The team member reinforces the statement by saying, "I'll make sure doctor looks at the tooth when she does her examination." The single-tooth syndrome builds steam during the examination as the dentist only looks for individual problems and only talks about individual solutions. The single-tooth syndrome climaxes at the treatment conference. The person presenting the case goes around the mouth one tooth at a time, tells the patient what needs to be done one tooth at a time, and then gives the patient a computer printout listing individual teeth, individual code numbers, and individual restorations needed.

The cure for the single tooth syndrome is simple: Talk to patients about comprehensive restorative solutions, not about individual teeth. As an example, at the before-the-examination conversation, if the patient says, "I have a broken metal filling on the upper right," respond with, "I'll make a note of that. Have you ever broken a metal filling or broken the tooth around a metal filling before?" Most people will reply, "Yes." Then ask, "How many other big metal fillings do you have in your mouth?" They may respond with, "Oh, I don't know. Three or four, I guess." You then say, "I'll make sure that when doctor does his exam he checks **all of them** for you."

Then, after the examination conversation is completed, sit the patient up and say, "Maria, you have five large, old metal fillings in your mouth. One is broken, one is decayed, and the other three are just worn out. The next time you come in, we'll discuss what we can do to take care of **all of them**."

At the solutions conversation, give the patients several great reasons why single-tooth dentistry is not in their best interest. As an example, "Maria, I mentioned last time that you have five large metal fillings that are decayed, broken, and just plain worn out. The best way to restore **these five teeth** is with tooth-colored restorations. We could do these five restorations one at a time. The problem with that is it takes two visits to do each restoration. That means you'd be coming in ten times. You'd have to take off work ten times. We'd have to numb up your mouth ten times. Plus, it's very difficult to make the color and shape of the restorations match if we do them one at a time. It's much better to do them all at once. That way we can do them in just three visits."

As you can see, the single-tooth syndrome has as much to do with your team's thinking and actions as it does with your patients' attitudes. From the very beginning, you must focus on comprehensive solutions, not individual teeth. When your whole team does this, the single-tooth syndrome will be cured in your office.

5. **Be like Columbo.** You may remember the *Columbo* television series that ran from 1971 through 1978. Lt. Columbo was a scruffy-looking, low-key cop who would never directly confront the suspects at first. He would just ask simple questions that would lead people to open up. Here's an example of the Columbo approach in a solutions conversation. If you have an idea that Maria may be overwhelmed by a fee you quote, tell her, "I know spending that much money may be completely out of the question for your family at this time. I certainly don't want to embarrass you. Maybe I shouldn't have mentioned the implants and veneers?"

If Maria says, "Yeah, that's a little much for our family right now," you can back off on the more comprehensive care. However, the majority of people will come to your defense at this point in time and say, "Oh, no. I want you to tell me about the best care." You reply, "Thanks for saying that." Then just keep going.

6. **Don't fry their brains.** If patients have to choose *what* care they desire and *how* they are going to pay for it with a single decision, their brains will fry. It's way too much information for them to process. Break their decision-making process into two parts. First have them decide *what* dental care they want. The good, better, best method is

an excellent way to do this. After they have decided *what* they want, they can choose *how* they want to pay for it. Your dental care agreement helps simplify the process for them by listing their four options.

7. **No knowledge of price = no true decision.** You would never make a decision to buy a specific model of car without knowing the price of the car. Likewise, don't put your patients in the position of agreeing to a care plan without knowing what their investment will be. The person presenting the good, better, and best care choices should also present the fees associated with each choice.

8. **Use the drop-down method if that is on brand for your office.** High-end offices may prefer to use the drop-down method. With it, you present *best* solutions only at first. Then drop down to *better* care if patients don't want to accept the best. This may also be the method of choice for patients who come in asking for the *best* care. After you present the *best* solution, ask, "Would you like to schedule your visits for this care?" If you have to drop down and present *better* care, ask, "Does this work better for you?"

9. **No pressure and no confusion.** At the solutions conversation, there should never be any pressure. You're there to serve them. They make the decisions that are best for them. There should be no confusion either. Have your good, better, and best plans and the investment options for each prepared ahead of time on your investment options agreements. Don't present solutions and then scramble around to calculate the investment options. Have your ducks in a row **before** the visit. PCC's have the time to do this.

Monitor Your Progress

On your practice management software, monitor your case-acceptance percentage for each month, each quarter, and the year-to-date. If you do this on paper, divide the total dollar amount of care accepted by patients during each time period by the total dollar amount of care your team presented to patients. As an example, if in the first quarter of 2013 you present $700,000 worth of care to patients and they accept $400,000, your case-acceptance percentage for that quarter is 57 percent. Here are two important points to remember about your case-acceptance percentage:

1. Most of the time, increasing the amount of comprehensive implant dentistry you present will lower your case-acceptance percentage. This is fine because the total amount of comprehensive dentistry accepted will increase.
2. Because all offices are different, don't compare your case-acceptance percentage with other offices. Focus on improving your percentage as you continue to offer patients the best implant dentistry possible.

Conclusion

This chapter has a plethora of information in a fairly compact form. You may want to re-read it before you move on to the next chapter on the fifth stage of creative case conversation, which is decision.

> *People who want milk should not seat themselves*
> *on a stool in the middle of a field*
> *in hopes that the cow will back up to them.*
>
> ELBERT HUBBARD

Take Elbert's advice and don't wait for the cow to back up to you. Make a smart decision now by reading the next chapter.

CHAPTER 15

Creative Case Conversation: Decision

IN THE LAST CHAPTER, you discovered how to present solutions to patients on the routine, foundational, and comprehensive care paths. At the end of the solutions conversation, you ask them how they want to proceed. The percentage of patients who say, "Yes," to one of the choices you give them depends on three factors:

1. **The type of people who are attracted to your office.** People who desire the dentistry you recommend are much more likely to accept your treatment plans. You don't have to push them. You just make it easy for them to receive the best that modern implant dentistry has to offer.

2. **The quality and type of dentistry you recommend.** If you only recommend low levels of care, the percentage of people who say, "Yes," increases. If you recommend comprehensive dentistry that includes implants when appropriate, the percentage of people who say, "Yes," decreases. And that's okay. Your case-acceptance percentage may go down, but people receive more of the highest quality care—and your net income goes up.

3. **Your skill in orchestrating creative case conversations.** These conversations are designed to help patients make a series of small,

easy, and comfortable steps to case acceptance. The conversations include, but are not limited to:

- the *marketing* conversation, where you create a brand that resonates with a certain group of people and they reach out to you via the web and/or phone.
- the *first phone call* conversation, when you begin to connect with them and they begin to connect with you.
- the *before-the- examination* conversation, in which you understand them as you learn their past, present, and future stories. They understand your office philosophy and the services you provide.
- the *examination* conversation, in which you and they become educated about their clinical condition in the gum and bone, restorative, replacement, and cosmetic areas.
- the *after-the-examination* conversation, when you and your patients on the comprehensive dentistry path have a general conversation about the possible care options. They inform you of the direction in which they would like to proceed.
- the *solutions* conversation, where you and they discuss specific solutions and financial options. They make the decisions that are best for them.
- *ongoing* conversations, when you ask people which solution works best for them, and they answer with some form of yes, no, or maybe. The ongoing conversations you have from that point will depend on their answers and the actions they take. This conversation may last for years.

In this chapter, you will learn how to effectively participate in these ongoing conversations, which are part of stage six of creative case conversation: decision.

Stage Six: Decision

You follow-up.
They follow through.

Stage six occurs after the solutions conversation. Although it would be wonderful if everyone made the decision to say, "Yes," to the comprehensive dentistry you propose in the solutions conversation, in reality people are going to say, "Yes," "No," or "Maybe."

1. **If they say, "Yes,"** congratulate them on their decision, have them sign the agreement, and schedule their appointments.

2. **If they say, "No,"** discover if the "no" means "no, never" or "no, not now." If they say, "No, I would never do comprehensive dentistry. I just want to patch things up when I have to," that means you haven't done an effective job of discovering their desires and pains in your previous conversations. It also means they may be happier in another dental office. If they say, "No, I can't do comprehensive dentistry now because of financial considerations," reply with, "I understand. Let's start the care that absolutely needs to be done. When your financial situation improves—at any time in the future—we'll be here for you."

3. **If they say, "Maybe,"** in the form of, "I want to think about it," or "I need to talk with my partner," or "I need to check our finances," you have three ways to respond:

    a. **Have them back for a final consultation.** Say, "I understand completely. Let's have you back for a final consultation with your partner. That way we answer all your questions so you can make an informed decision." Or, "I understand completely. Let's call your partner and see if we can get him/her in to help you both make an informed decision."

    b. **Set a decision date.** Say, "I understand. When do you think you will make your decision?" They give you a date. Then say, "If we haven't heard from you by (a day after the date they told you), is it okay if I give you a call? I want to make sure we get started with your gum and bone therapy/fix that broken tooth/start that root canal."

c. **Get started with something.** If they continue to put off making a decision on comprehensive care, get them appointed for their most urgent care, such as perio therapy, a badly broken tooth, or a root canal. Don't let the "Maybe" people just float away. Get started with something. After you do, and they experience your level of care, they may want to proceed with comprehensive care.

Ongoing Conversations

People like Maria who don't make the decision to have *all* their comprehensive dentistry quickly completed will end up in your recare system. At their recare visits, your hygienists will be primarily responsible for having the ongoing creative case conversations with them. Here are three questions that effectively start the conversations.

1. "Have you heard or read anything about dentistry that you would like to know more about?"

2. "Maria, last year you had two of your worst metal fillings replaced with tooth-colored restorations. There are three more metal fillings in your mouth that should be replaced as soon as possible. What are your thoughts about doing them at this time?" Identify any forces that may be limiting their action. If possible, work through these limiting forces.

3. Wait for a significant change in the patient's condition (another broken filling, continued loss of bone, or drifting of teeth) as your opening to talk about recommended care again. As an example, "Maria, the lower partial denture that the doctor made for you two years ago is as strong as ever. But the bone supporting it is continuing to melt away. That's why the partial is rocking a little just like the first one did. This is also putting some extra pressure on those two teeth the partial is attached to. Have you given any more thought to having implants on the lower? I know your upper implant is doing great."

If Maria responds that she has given it some thought, respond with, "Great, let's talk with the doctor when he comes in to see you in a few minutes."

Quadrant Dentistry Is Nice

What would happen to your bottom line if you could do 50 percent more quadrant dentistry than you're doing right now? How much time and hassle could you save your patients? The answers to both questions are, "A lot." Here's how it can happen.

At a recare visit, your well-trained hygienist sees that Shirley's tooth #3 has a fractured amalgam. She also sees that teeth #2 and #4 are restored with large amalgams that have seen better days. She says to the patient, "Shirley, take a look on the screen. You have one metal filling that is fractured. It definitely needs to be restored as soon as possible with a tooth-colored restoration. Do you see the teeth in front of and behind the tooth with the fractured filling? The fillings in those teeth have been in your mouth a long time. Those fillings are crumbling around the edges. There is also a crack on the cheek side of the back tooth. If you have those three teeth restored one at a time, it will take six visits. You'll have to take off work six times and have your mouth numbed six times. If we do all three at once, it will only take two visits. Would you like to explore the possibility of doing all three? I think the doctor might recommend tooth-colored onlays and crowns. We can talk with her about it when she comes in?"

"Would You Like to Explore the Possibility of...?"

I've seen it happen on numerous occasions. A dentist goes to a conference and hears a consultant proclaim, "Your hygienists need to sell quadrant dentistry. Give them a financial incentive for doing so. If they don't want to sell, give them a career redirection opportunity." The dentist comes back to the real world, puts pressure on his hygienist to sell, and unveils his new and improved compensation system—only to create a situation where the hygienist angrily leaves the practice.

The process doesn't have to go like that. I hope you have an office full of hygienists who love to close cases. Even if you don't, I'm offering you a way to help your hygienists be more effective right now at making it easy for patients to accept comprehensive dentistry. The secret lies in the question, "Would you like to explore the possibility of...?"

In the example above, the hygienist asked, "Would you like to explore the possibility of doing all three? I think the doctor might recommend tooth-colored onlays and crowns. We can talk with her about it when she comes in." The "Would you like to explore the possibility of…?" question accomplishes two outcomes:

1. It comfortably guides the patient toward quadrant dentistry. She doesn't make the final decision. She just takes a small step in that direction.

2. It's less threatening to the hygienist. She's not selling. She's offering an opportunity for education and a choice.

This same question can be used by your team in other situations. As an example, a patient mentions to your clinical assistant that she doesn't like the appearance of her front teeth. Your well-trained and alert assistant says, "Gertrude, you can have a beautiful smile in only two visits by having veneers done. Take a look at some of these before and after pictures of cases like yours that doctor has done. Would you like to explore the possibility of doing the same? We can talk to him about it when he comes in."

There are dozens of times when everyone in the office can help patients move forward with care using the "Would you like to explore the possibility of…?" question. Have a team meeting to discuss possibilities and then role-play the specific situations.

The Handoff to the Doctor

In the sample quadrant conversation, the hygienist asked the patient, "Would you like to explore the possibility of doing all three? I think the doctor might recommend tooth-colored onlays and crowns. We can talk with her about it when she comes in."

If the patient says, "Yes," here's how the hygienist should do the handoff to the doctor. "Doctor, Shirley has a fractured filling on her upper right first molar. The teeth in front of and behind the tooth with the fractured filling have metal fillings that are worn out. I've shown Shirley how the edges of the fillings are crumbling and how one of the teeth has a crack on the cheek side. I told Shirley you would probably recommend tooth-colored restorations on those three teeth. Shirley said she would like to explore the possibility of doing all three at once. Take a look and tell us what you think."

Have a Toolbox Full of Patient Stories

When you have a toolbox full of stories, you can pull out the best one at the right time when you're having ongoing conversations with a patient. The best stories are those concerning other patients who had dental problems similar to the troubles this person is having. Each story should have four parts.

1. the other patient's dental problem and how it was affecting her life
2. the action the other patient took to solve the problem
3. the positive results the other patient received by taking the action
4. the transference of the story's message to the person you're speaking with

Here's an example of this type of conversation: "Bruce, I know making the decision to have implants on the bottom and having a snap-in denture is a big one. You've been wearing that old lower denture for a long time and it's hard to make a decision to change sometimes. Can I tell you a story about one of our other patients? Max is about your age and, like you, had a lower denture that floated all over the place. He couldn't eat with it and only wore it when he had to. We talked about doing implants and a snap-in denture for three or four years. Finally he decided to take the leap of faith a year ago.

"He absolutely loves his new denture. He leaves it in all day and eats whatever he wants. Look at these before and after photos of his face. It looks like he's ten years younger, doesn't it? We have dozens of patients just like Max. They've all made the decision to have implants. And they all tell me the same thing, 'I wish I would have done it sooner.' Bruce, I'm sure you will tell me the same thing when you have your new snap-in denture."

Use Analogies Well

When explaining concepts to patients, an excellent strategy is to use analogies. They're a great way of showing patients how something they already understand is similar to something you would like them to understand. Here's an example: "Those four old metal fillings in your mouth are like worn-out tires on your car. Some people replace their tires when the tread is low. Some people replace them when the tread is worn smooth. Some people replace them after a tire blows out. Most of my patients don't want to be stranded with a dental blowout. It's up to you. We can replace those fillings now with tooth-colored restorations, or we can wait for something bad to happen. The choice is yours."

Conclusion

Decision is the sixth stage of creative case conversation, and the content and tone of your ongoing conversations with patients are heavily influenced by your team's attitudes towards the completion of comprehensive dentistry. If you don't firmly believe comprehensive dentistry is in your patients' best interests, you won't talk to them about it or will talk about it in half-hearted ways. The same goes for your team: they need to believe it to convey it.

If you do firmly believe comprehensive dentistry is in your patients' best interests, you will talk to them about it in respectful ways. Need some evidence to support this belief? I'm sure you have several instances of patients putting off comprehensive care for three, four, or five years and then finally taking action. Aren't they always glad the care was completed? In fact, don't they always say, "I wish I would have done this sooner"?

When you approach patients with the "They will be glad they did it when all is said and done" attitude, you will say the right words in the right way with the right body language… and your patients will definitely get the message.

Another time you will want to have belief behind your words is when you discuss money. In the next chapter, you will learn how to have money discussions early, often, and comfortably in a process I call massaging money magnificently. Intrigued? Read on.

CHAPTER 16

Massage Money Magnificently

IN MOST DENTAL PRACTICES, who among the team likes talking about money with patients? Clinical assistants? Nope. Hygienists? Not usually. Dentists? You've got to be kidding. In most offices, the only people who enjoy discussing money are good financial coordinators.

So any time patients ask a question even remotely dealing with money, in a traditional practice the clinical assistants, hygienists, and doctors employ one of their two well-rehearsed escape mechanisms. They say:

1. "I don't know," when they do know or have a general idea, or
2. "Our financial coordinator, Judy, will explain all that to you later."

After escaping the dreaded M-word conversation, they think, "Whew! I almost had to talk about money there." So what's the result of this ongoing evasion? The discussion of money is perpetually delayed until it pops up (explodes may be a better choice of words) at the end of the treatment conference.

Here's an example of what I mean. Milton is a patient in Dr. Avoidit's office. Milton needs several implants and accompanying restorative dentistry. He is treated extremely well by everyone in the office. At the first visit, the doctor does a thorough examination. Milton sees a very impressive video on the advantages of implant dentistry and the various types of implants available. He's excited to return for the treatment conference in a week.

At the treatment conference, Dr. Avoidit does a masterful job of presenting the very best implant care available. Milton is even more enthused now. He says to the doctor, "Looks great, doc. How much is all this going to cost?"

Dr. Avoidit immediately selects escape mechanism #2 (his personal favorite) and replies, "Our financial coordinator, Judy, will explain all that to you in just a few minutes." He then wipes the sweat off his brow and does a flawless hand-off to Judy as she enters the room.

Judy is a very pleasant and extremely knowledgeable financial coordinator. She asks if Milton has any questions about the treatment the doctor recommended. Milton answers, "Just how much the dentistry is going to cost."

Judy captures a gulp of air and proudly announces, "The fee to do all your implant and restorative dentistry is $23,700." There is silence in the room as Milton tries to get a grasp on the figure. Judy is wondering how she's going to do the financial arrangements and CPR at the same time.

Milton mutters, "Boy, that's a lot more than I thought it would be. My insurance will cover most of it, right?"

Judy proclaims, "I'm afraid your insurance will only cover $1,000."

Is Milton in the frame of mind to make a decision right after he has been figuratively hit over the head a couple of times with a baseball bat? He's dazed, disappointed, and discouraged. So he gathers his thoughts and replies, "I'm going to have to think about it."

Two weeks have gone by now. No one has heard from Milton. One day, Dr. Avoidit stops Judy in the hallway and says, "When's Milton coming in to get started? He was really excited to get going when I was with him. What happened?"

Judy feels like saying, "Nobody in this office would talk with Milton about money, financing, and insurance early so I had to whack him over the head with a baseball bat at the worst possible time. He was nice about it, but we'll probably never see him again." Instead Judy is more tactful and says, "Milton is still thinking about it."

I'm guessing there are hundreds of Miltons in your practice right now who are "thinking about it." What a shame. They aren't getting the care that will enhance their lives and you aren't receiving the income that will improve your bottom line.

Four Vital Case Acceptance Understandings

In Chapter 11, you learned that you and your patients need to understand each other for comprehensive case acceptance to progress. There are four vital case acceptance understandings that all your patients should have after specific care has been discussed:

Understanding #1: "I knew they were going to discuss comprehensive care." Unless they instruct you differently, one of your treatment options should be the best that dentistry has to offer.

Understanding #2: "The fee is about what I thought it would be." If you were shopping in a clothing store and saw an interesting item, what would you do before trying it on? You'd look at the price tag, wouldn't you? The same is true of your patients. Before mentally "trying on" dental care, your patients need to know approximately what it will cost them monetarily.

Understanding #3: "I know I can finance all or part of my investment in dental care. I'm already approved. I don't have to pay for all of this at once." As the Milton story illustrates, if you begin to discuss finances only after you present the good, better, and best treatment options, you whack people with a club and lose all your momentum.

Understanding #4: "I'm in control of what we do now. They're here to suggest options and serve my wishes." It's vital that everyone is clear on their roles in the case conversation process. You are the consultants who serve. The patients are the decision-makers who are in control.

The above four understandings take place when your team learns to talk about money early in the conversations you have with patients. I call this process "massaging money." To effectively massage money your team needs to:
- maintain empowering beliefs about financing
- choose the best financing partner
- have a variety of ways to discuss money and financing.

Seven Empowering Beliefs about Financing

Limiting beliefs lead to actions that hold you back in your practice—and your life. Empowering beliefs lead to actions that move you forward. From my discussions with hundreds of successful dentists, I've identified seven empowering beliefs they consistently hold about patient financing:

Belief #1: It is professional to offer financing for dental care. In the past five years, I've seen dentists' attitudes change on this one. An increasing number of dentists have come to realize that their competition isn't the dentist *across* the street. It's the Best Buy store *down* the street. I can guarantee you Best Buy offers financing (many times no-interest financing) on most purchases. The question you need to answer is, "Is the dental care we provide just as important as a new flat screen television?" If the answer is, "Yes," then you need to believe in offering financing in your office.

Belief #2: I can't really know who's going to accept financing, so I offer it to everybody. It's virtually impossible to tell which of your patients need financing. Many patients are embarrassed to ask about financing and won't discuss it unless you bring it up. In addition, it's difficult to tell which patients will choose to receive a 5 percent accounting reduction and pay for their care up front. Assume everyone is a candidate for financing. Assume everyone is a candidate for paying in advance. Offer both options to everyone. Doing so will increase case acceptance rates by 10 to 25 percent.

Belief #3: Offering no-interest financing for dental care doesn't cost me money. It saves me money. At the end of the month, some dentists look at how much it cost them to do business with the no-interest finance company. They would be better served by seeing how financing added to their bottom line in the following ways:

- You will do fewer removable partial dentures and more dental implants. The amount you net per hour on implants is vastly higher than your reward for spending an hour with members of the partial denture club.

- You won't be the bank. It doesn't pay. If your patients have 36 different kinds of bills to pay, you will be 35 on the list. The average dental office collects 96 percent of their production. That's 4 percent that wouldn't be lost if you used financing and got paid the day you started your procedures.

- You won't send as many (or any) statements. Numerous studies have shown it costs you $10 per statement sent. How many do you send each month? Multiply that times $10.
- Your patients won't get the checkbook chills. Here's what I mean: It's Monday evening. Your patient, Steve, sees he has an appointment scheduled for the next day to seat a crown. He knows he must bring in a check for $600. He looks in his checkbook and notices his balance is $132.27. Steve begins to shiver and comes down with a bad case of the checkbook chills. He calls your office at midnight, informs you of his condition, and says he will call you when he's feeling better. The moral of the story: Don't combine an office visit with a payment. They don't mix well.

Belief #4: Money is the problem. Have you ever heard a dental practice management guru say, "When it comes to case acceptance, money isn't the real problem. If you build enough value for the care, people will consistently say, 'Yes,' to your treatment plans." I'm certainly in favor of building value for dental care, but there are limits. Statistics show at least 60 percent of patients are unwilling or unable to accept treatment plans because of financial constraints. Just accept that money *is* the problem and follow the suggestions in this chapter to lessen its effect.

Belief #5: I'm booked solid now. I can be booked more effectively with patient financing. Some offices don't use financing because they're booked solid now. I'm guessing they're booked solid with lots of small restorative procedures causing everyone to frantically rush around the office trying to keep up. With patient financing, you will be booked solid with longer visits involving more high-end dentistry.

Belief #6: Phasing care can be more expensive for my patients. When it comes to financing, realize that patients are going to *pay* for their comprehensive care over time whether they finance their care and have it all done immediately or if they phase their care. If they finance their care with a no-interest plan, it can be *less expensive* for them to have everything done now because the cost of care will increase each year and they'll experience fewer emergency situations. In other words, phasing care can be more expensive for your patients than financing!

Belief #7: Financing leads to better relationships with our patients. Have you ever been to a resort destination or on a week-long cruise where you pay an all-inclusive fee before you check in? It's neat, isn't it? Now you can enjoy your vacation without thinking about money. A similar reaction occurs when your patients don't have to pay at every visit.

That's not the only reason financing improves relationships. In general, what do people think of those to whom they owe money? There's often a weird form of resentment felt each time the borrower writes a check. And if the borrower is late with payments, it puts a strain on the relationship and on both parties, doesn't it?

> *The holy passion of friendship is of so sweet and steady and loyal and enduring a nature that it will last through a whole lifetime, if not asked to lend money.*
>
> MARK TWAIN

Now that you have your empowering patient financing beliefs in place, it's time to choose the best financing partner.

Selecting the Best Financing Partner

The decision concerning who will be the best financing partner for your practice is one of the most important management choices you will ever make. I purposely use the term financing *partner*. You need to work together to help more patients receive the care they deserve.

Here are nine questions you can use to evaluate financing partners:

1. **Do they offer generous credit lines?** Every credit approval should have a minimum credit line of $5,000. Any amount less than that will severely hinder your case conversation process.

2. **Do they have high approval rates?** Different finance companies use varying criteria to judge the credit-worthiness of patients. After using a new financing partner for a period of time, you will be able to see how their approval rates compare with your current financing partner.

3. **Do they offer a revolving line of credit at locked-in interest rates?** Choose a financing partner that offers a revolving line of credit so additional treatment fees can easily be added in the future. The interest rate should also be locked in and not tied to a fluctuating prime rate.

4. **Do they offer no-interest financing for as long as 24 months?** No-interest financing is hugely popular with consumers and very affordable. Financing $9,000 worth of care for 24 months is only about $378 a month. One of the fastest-growing patient-financing companies reports that over 80 percent of its customers choose no-interest financing. For maximum effectiveness, offer your patients no-interest and extended payment plans.

5. **Do they offer no-interest finance plans with equal monthly payments?** This question is more important than it may seem. Some finance companies offer extremely low (usually 3 percent of the balance) with a huge balloon payment at the end. As you might imagine, the balloon method will create an unwelcome surprise to some of your patients who only make the minimum payments.

   To illustrate what I mean, imagine that on a 12-month no-interest balloon plan, only 11.3 percent of the amount financed is paid in the first 11 months if minimum payments are made. That leaves 88.7 percent due on the 12th month. On an $8,000 loan, $7,096 must be paid or the no-interest plan turns into a traditional extended pay plan with interest accruing every month at annual rates of over 20 percent! And who do you think is going to get a phone call when the patient's 12th month statement comes with all this cheery information? You will—and the call won't be a pleasant one.

   On a $2,400, 12-month, no-interest, equal monthly payment plan, patients pay back $2,400 in principal and interest in 12 months if they regularly pay on time. On a $2,400 balloon payment plan, if patients only make the minimum payments each month (very tempting for some people), they will pay back $6,250.46 in 19 years and seven months! Moral to the story: don't mess with balloon payment plans.

6. **Do they offer case conversation tools?** Customized case conversation tools such as the payment options worksheet will save you time and make it easier for people to say, "Yes."

7. **Do they have an online reporting and tracking service?** The service should allow you to view your transactions in real time 24/7 via the Internet. Don't wait for a monthly report of patient financing activity. The service should also allow you to track individual patient applications, approvals, and confirmation of payment as well as generate daily-updated reports of all outstanding approvals for the past 90 days.

8. **Do they work with your practice management software provider?** Choose a partner that will work with your practice management software company to install an interface allowing you to apply for patient financing using the existing information in your files. This will allow you to pre-qualify a patient in seconds, while you're on the phone with them.

9. **Do they provide extensive ongoing training?** Choose a company that will help you integrate the system into your practice and provide evaluations after implementation.

Learn a Variety of Ways to Discuss Money and Financing

Now that you have your empowering patient financing beliefs in place and the best financing partner selected, it's time to identify the times and ways you can discuss money and financing. Before you do this, it's important to keep in mind that patient financing is more of an art than a science. Your success is dependent on the styles and personalities of the people in your office. Your entire team needs to believe in the principle of patient financing. If you have people who don't believe in patient financing, they should be put in positions where they don't have financing conversations with patients—or they should be given career adjustments.

When discussing financing with patients, your team should be coming from the right place in their hearts. They are not takers. They never press the issue. They are givers who are here to serve people by giving them additional options that will allow them to receive the best dental care sooner.

Here are 16 opportunities and methods you can use to discuss money and financing. **Don't use all 16 with every patient.** That would be way too much information discussed way too often. Just pull out the best method at the right time from your handy dandy massaging money methods toolbox. In addition, make sure the use of each method is on brand for your practice.

1. Mention that "No-Interest Financing Options Are Available" in your internal and external marketing.

2. Have a link from your website to your finance partner's application page on their website. Do not link it to their homepage because there is probably a "search for a dentist" link on it with names and addresses of other dentists in your area.

3. On your website, have a page that reviews the payment options you make available.

4. On the first phone call, if they bring up a money issue or inquire about financing, briefly explain your no-interest payment plans and then invite them to the office.

5. On the first phone call, if they are price shoppers, follow the script in Chapter 10: Fantastic Phone Fundamentals.

6. As part of the new patient packet you send out between the first phone call and the first visit—if they've asked about financing, brought up a money issue, or appear to be a shopper—mail or e-mail them the mailed welcome letter in Appendix A.

7. At the first visit, if they've asked about financing, brought up a money issue, or given the impression of being a shopper, give them the in-office welcome letter in Appendix A as part of your new patient information material.

8. If at anytime during the first visit they ask about financing or bring up a money issue, answer by saying, "I appreciate you bringing that up. If you want to, we can get you pre-approved with our financing partner ahead of time. That way we will have a plan in place where you can spread out the investment in your dentistry if you desire." Then, give them the in-office welcome letter and explain your financing options.

9. Remember Question #10 in the office conversation before the dental exam: "Is there anything that would stand in your way of getting the proper dentistry you need?" If they mention that money could be a problem, immediately give them the in-office welcome letter and explain your financing options.

10. For patients on the comprehensive and foundational care paths, care is discussed in general in a conversation after the exam. For these patients, give them the in-office welcome letter and explain your financing options—but no specifics yet.

11. When you quote fees for patients on the comprehensive and foundational care paths at the second visit and for the patients on the routine care path at the first visit, follow the quote of a fee with what their monthly payments would be for the good, better, and best options. As an example, "Maria, the fee to complete the dentistry we just discussed is $9,000, or $378 a month if you want to spread it out over time with our no-interest financing plan."

12. After patients on the comprehensive care path choose the good, better, or best care option they desire, use the financing options worksheet as a tool to discuss their payment choices. If they choose a no-interest payment plan or an extended pay plan, go ahead and apply for financing now. (Remember, this is almost the worst time to do this. It's much better to bring up financing at the times indicated in the previous 11 methods.)

13. If patients are declined for financing, encourage them to reapply with a cosigner.

14. Follow up with your "maybe" patients on the phone. If appropriate, offer again to help them with financing their care.

15. If you are new to no-interest financing, send a follow-up letter similar to the one in Appendix A to "maybe" patients who've been presented care in the past year but didn't schedule visits. Statistics show that 60 percent didn't schedule because of financial considerations.

16. At recare visits, offer your financing options to patients who have uncompleted or newly identified care.

Quote Comprehensive Fees with Confidence

It's vital that the people quoting your comprehensive fees are comfortable doing so. If they aren't, all the right *words* may be said, but their voice qualities and body language are saying, "I don't feel comfortable doing this." Or worse, "I don't really think you should spend this much money on dentistry."

If a member of your team isn't comfortable with quoting fees, you have three choices: (1) don't have them do it; (2) give them a new career opportunity; or (3) show them how everyone wins with comprehensive dentistry.

At your team meetings, frequently tell stories of patients who delayed doing their comprehensive care for three or four years and then finally had it completed. How often do they say, "I wish we hadn't done this?" Almost never, right? In fact, don't they almost always say, "I wish we would have done this sooner." Don't be afraid to diagnose and present comprehensive care with high fees. You're doing everyone a favor.

Conclusion

The information in the last four chapters is simple information. You just answer the phone fantastically, guide people through the six stages of creative case conversations, and then massage money magnificently. But *simple* isn't always *easy* to do. It may require your team and you to change some beliefs. It may require you to change your systems. You may make some mistakes. Some team members may dislike what you're doing at first, but they will love it when they see the results.

> *Our dilemma is that we hate change*
> *and love it at the same time;*
> *what we really want is for things*
> *to remain the same but get better.*
>
> SYDNEY HARRIS

Sydney is right. For things to get better for everyone, you must take the first step of building a solid practice foundation. Next you must become a master marketer. Then you must make it easy for people to accept comprehensive implant dentistry. Now that you have done these three, you must take the next step and keep your promises. Start now. Promise you will turn this page and continue reading.

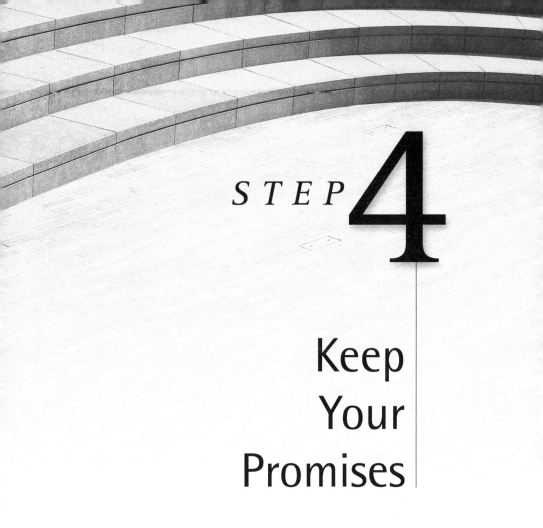

STEP 4

Keep Your Promises

THE FIRST STEP ON YOUR JOURNEY TO IMPLANT EXCELLENCE is to build a solid practice foundation with the four cornerstones of dreams, character, team, and branding. The second step is to become a master marketer by marketing internally to your current patients, marketing externally to your community, and using public relations to shine a positive light on your practice. The third step is to make it easy for people to accept the comprehensive implant dentistry you love to do.

Now you're ready for Step 4: keeping your promises. Back in Chapter 4, you discovered that your brand consists of the words, images, and emotions that are stored in the minds of the people in your community, and your patients in particular. At one time, Tiger Woods was this brand: "A golfer who combines natural talent, hard work, and enthusiasm to be a champion and role model for all ages and ethnicities." That was a terrific brand making Tiger millions of dollars. Unfortunately for all of us, Tiger broke his promise. He not only lost millions, but he lost respect and his wife. Moral: Don't make a brand promise and then break it. You're better off not making the promise in the first place.

Just like Tiger, your brand is the promise you make to the community concerning what to expect when they come to your office. Congratulations! You've just put yourself on the hot seat. Now you've got to deliver on your promises by providing on-brand clinical excellence and staging memorable experiences. The two chapters in this section will show you how to do that, and live up to your brand.

CHAPTER 17

Provide Clinical Excellence

Once there was a successful company that manufactured and sold shoes. One day the management had a meeting to consider selling their shoes in the faraway country of Babushka. They sent one of their top salespersons to the country to study its market potential. Immediately upon arriving, he noticed that almost all of the people were barefooted. He e-mailed home the message, "Bad news, nobody wears shoes here!" He followed up with a detailed report explaining why no market for shoes existed in Babushka.

The management wanted to get a second opinion, so they sent another salesperson to Babushka. Upon her arrival, the second salesperson was so excited she quickly e-mailed a message back, "Good news, nobody wears shoes here!" She hurried home and reported to the management, "Gentlemen, we're going to be rich. There's a monster market in Babushka. All we need to do is educate Babushkans on how wearing shoes will be to their advantage."

This story illustrates that life is how you perceive it. There's a negative side and a positive side to every practice situation. If you have a doughnut, you can choose to either look at the hole, or look at the dough. The choice is yours.

> *We don't see things as they are.*
> *We see things as we are.*
>
> ANAIS NIN

I relate the shoe story because I sometimes meet dentists who tell me, "I'd love to take your *implant courses* and do the comprehensive implant dentistry you teach, but people in my area just aren't interested." That comment sounds like the first salesperson, doesn't it?

In this chapter, you will learn all about the following four keys to providing clinical excellence:

1. Attend comprehensive surgical and/or restorative implant training programs with hands-on training
2. Create and communicate your implant philosophy
3. Receive informed consent before surgery
4. Schedule for clinical excellence

Key #1: Attend comprehensive surgical and/or restorative implant training programs with hands-on training.

Your best bet is to enroll in a market-leading program that has an experienced team of lecturers. Be sure the program is noncommercial—not one taught or hosted by an implant company or by a person with strong ties or financial relationships to a single implant company. Be sure the program director is approachable before, during, and after the program for questions and concerns which might arise on your educational journey. I know I'm a little biased, but I believe the hands-on live-patient programs we offer at Implant Seminars are the best trainings available today.

> *Live as if you were to die tomorrow.*
> *Learn as if you were to live forever.*
> MAHATMA GANDHI

Key #2: Create and communicate your implant philosophy.

It's vital that you create an individual philosophy concerning the placement and restoration of implants, and then communicate your beliefs to your team. The philosophy should include *who, why, what, when, where,* and *how* components:

- **Who:** Who do I consider as candidates for implants?
- **Why:** Why do these people need the implants done? Include the consequences for not having the surgery completed and the benefits that will be obtained with implants.
- **What:** What types of implants do we place for the who's and why's above?
- **When:** When do we place the implants? Are there any procedures that must be finished before the implants are placed? When are the fixed and removable prostheses completed?
- **Where:** Where do our implant patients come from? What percent are new patients? What percent are existing patients? What percent are referrals from other dentists?
- **How:** How do we place the implants and construct the fixed and removable prostheses?

After you create your implant philosophy, communicate it to your entire team. Show them cases you've completed. Review the who, why, what, when, where, and how with each case. Then show your team some other cases and have your team tell you what they believe the who, why, what, when, where, and how will be with each case.

Your implant philosophy will change as existing technologies—and your skills—improve. Update your beliefs yearly and communicate your changes to the team.

Key #3: Receive informed consent before surgery.

It's vital that you obtain informed consent before you perform any kind of implant surgery. You will need forms for extractions, gingival grafting surgery, guided tissue augmentation, dental implants, augmentation grafting of maxillary sinus, and sinus elevation with immediate implant placement.

Each form should have the following legal subject headings:

- condition
- procedure
- alternatives
- consequences of not having the procedure
- risks
- drugs, medication, and anesthesia
- implant database
- no guarantee
- my responsibility
- necessary follow-up care and self-care
- photography
- miscellaneous
- fees understanding

I recommend you obtain informed consent forms that include all of the above topics. The forms should be written by medical lawyers and updated regularly. The informed consent documents on CD from ImplantVision (www.implantvision.net) are the best I've found.

Key #4: Schedule for clinical excellence.

Your schedule can control you, or you can control your schedule. The choice is yours. When you're in charge, everything will improve, from the quality of your clinical dentistry, to your patients' experiences, to your team's lives—as well as your bottom line. Here is my checklist for creating and implementing an effective procedure-based schedule.

1. Your schedule should reflect your practice philosophy concerning the percentage of the time you want to run on schedule, the degree of clinical excellence you want to give, and the memorable experiences you want to provide.

2. There are three basic types of schedules. A **single column schedule** works for one doctor, one clinical assistant, and one treatment room. This type of schedule creates very low stress for everyone, but leads to periods of doctor inactivity. The **double or triple column schedule** involves one doctor, two or more clinical assistants, and two or more treatment rooms. This schedule creates a hurried doctor, stressed team, and a collection of unhappy patients brooding in the "waiting room." The **procedure-based schedule** is the one I recommend for most offices. Involving one doctor, two clinical assistants, and two treatment rooms, this schedule creates low stress for everyone, maximum team productivity, and happy patients. I will explain the system for creating a procedure-based schedule shortly.

3. Assign two time periods for each procedure you typically perform. The first period is the patient's chair time, which equals the entire time the patient is in the office. The second time period is the amount of time the doctor is with the patient. Clinical assistants are the best people to do this. The assistants should time each procedure on three occasions and then calculate the average time. Doctors should not do this as they think almost every procedure takes less time than it actually does. The clinical assistant should covertly time you on three occasions for each clinical procedure and then calculate the average time period per procedure.

    To properly determine true patient chair time, the assistant calculates when she is in the room with the patient and when you are in the room together. When determining chair time, it's not just the time you have your hands in the patient's mouth. Chair time includes the patient's entire period in the office.

4. If the office is open four days a week, think of your week as four empty buckets. In each bucket, you will be placing *rocks*, *pebbles*, and *sand* procedures. *Rock* procedures are the higher investment ones, in

the $1,200 range (for example, indirect restorations and implants). *Pebble* procedures are ones in the $300 range (think of fillings and extractions). *Sand* procedures are those with no charge billed that day (stage II implant surgeries, seating crowns and making denture adjustments). If you don't save room for your rocks, the pebbles and sand will quickly fill your buckets. Without room for the rocks, your schedule will be full and you will be busy, but with a bucket full of pebbles and sand you probably won't reach your daily production goal.

If you have a daily production goal of $6,000, ask yourself this question, "Based on our fee schedule, how many rocks and pebbles do I need to put in each bucket to reach our daily production goal of $6,000?" For many dental offices, the answer is "four rocks and four pebbles." Using the information in the section of this book on making it easy for people, you should be getting your four rocks from one or two patients, not four patients. The same is true with your pebbles patients—one or two patients providing you with four pebbles.

5. **Do *not* schedule according to time.** An example of this would be scheduling a patient who needs 45 minutes to place two composite fillings in the next available 90-minute opening in your traditional schedule without considering the fact that you could use that opening to begin a "rock" procedure. ***Do* schedule according to procedure.** An example of this would be giving the patient who needs 45 minutes for two composite fillings the choice between the next two available blocks that you have pre-designated as pebbles.

6. Be sure the blocks of time set aside for your rocks, pebbles, and sand add up to your daily production goals for the doctor *and* each hygienist.

7. Using one of your blank schedules, create a procedure-based schedule template for an ideal day. Remember, you will schedule to this template. In the sample template below, there are three columns. Column one is doctor with clinical assistant #1 in treatment room #1. Column two is doctor with clinical assistant #2 in treatment

room #2. Column three is the hygienist. If you have a patient care coordinator who is with your new patients their entire first visit, she should have her own column. She doesn't need a separate treatment room.

SAMPLE PROCEDURE-BASED SCHEDULE

Monday, December 8

Time	ROOM #1	ROOM #2	ROOM #3
8 AM		Rock	Perio Therapy
9 AM	New Patient		Recare
10 AM	Pebble	Pebble	New Patient
11 AM	Emergency	Sand	Recare
12 PM	LUNCH	LUNCH	LUNCH
1 PM		Rock	Perio Therapy
2 PM	New Patient		Recare
3 PM	Pebble	Pebble	New Patient
4 PM	Emergency	Sand	Recare
5 PM			

In the procedure-based template above, notice that the doctor has a two-hour rock block of time from 8 to 10 am. A new patient comes in at 9 am to be with clinical assistant #1 for one hour. During the last 30 minutes of that hour, the doctor will see the new patient. The new patient then sees the hygienist for the last hour of the two-hour first visit. The hygienist has periodontal therapy blocks from 8 to 9 am and from 1 to 2 pm. This was purposely done so the doctor will not have a hygiene exam during the first hour of the doctor's rock blocks.

The doctor has three one-hour pebble blocks during the day as well as two one-hour sand blocks. The hygienist has two one-hour periodontal therapy blocks during the day, a single one-hour new patient block, and five one-hour recare blocks. Notice that the recare blocks are during the doctor's pebble and sand blocks so the doctor can spend five minutes doing the recare exams.

8. At your morning meetings, discuss rock blocks that are open in the next ten office days and your plan to fill them.

9. Any rock block three office days into the future that is not scheduled should be filled with pebble patients from your list of people who have pebble visits scheduled and have indicated they'd be willing to come in sooner on short notice.

10. Attracting ten to 16 quality new patients per month is ideal for most practices. This averages out to about one new patient per day.

11. Have two different procedure-based templates that you use during the week. Template #1 is used on Mondays and Wednesdays. Template two is used on Tuesdays and Thursdays. This will provide a choice of times during the day for your rock, pebble, and sand patients.

12. When scheduling patients, never ask, "When would you like to come in?" or "What time would be good for you?" This creates situations where the schedule controls you. Simply ask, "Doctor has Monday at 8:00 or Thursday at 2:00. Which works best for you?"

Conclusion

> *The secret of joy in work is contained*
> *in one word—excellence.*
> *To know how to do something well*
> *is to enjoy it.*
>
> PEARL S. BUCK

In this chapter, you learned four keys to providing clinical excellence. Of course, your patients are the prime beneficiaries of your excellent dentistry. And as Pulitzer- and Nobel Prize-winning American author Pearl S. Buck points out, you're a winner too. Your team *and* you receive the emotional and financial rewards that accompany excellence. Many dentists are mediocre. They earn a mediocre living doing mediocre dentistry on patients who think mediocre is fine, too. How much joy is wrapped up with that package?

> *Great spirits have always encountered*
> *violent opposition from mediocre minds.*
> *The mediocre mind is incapable of understanding*
> *the man who refuses to bow blindly*
> *to conventional prejudices*
> *and chooses instead to express his opinions*
> *courageously and honestly.*
>
> ALBERT EINSTEIN

The sad truth is that excellence makes people nervous. On your journey to excellence, there will be an army of people whose nervousness will propel them to resist you. The insurance companies don't like excellence. They only want to pay for mediocre dentistry. Your dental colleagues may not like it, because your clinical excellence shines a revealing beacon on their mediocrity. Your team may feel nervous about implementing some of your grand ideas. In the last section of this book, you will learn how to deal with all these nervous people.

One word of caution here: in your quest for excellence, don't try to be perfect. Perfection is a one-way street with a dead end. Doctors new to implant dentistry who try to be the perfect implant dentist will do one of two things: (1) they will never place their first new implant because they have established an impossible goal; or (2) they will place the implant, but fiddle with it so much trying to be perfect that they will lower the quality of the implant. When it comes to perfection, heed Michael J. Fox's words below:

*I am careful not to confuse excellence with perfection.
Excellence, I can reach for;
Perfection is God's business.*

MICHAEL J. FOX

Now that you've discovered how to keep your promises to patients with your clinical dentistry (*what* you do), it's time to keep your promises to them in the experiences you provide (*how* you do it). Turn the page now. The next few minutes will be a memorable experience for you.

CHAPTER 18

Stage Memorable Experiences

THERE'S A TYPE OF TELEVISION COMMERCIAL that has been running for decades. The first ad like this was for Folgers instant coffee. In one, an affluent couple is shown sipping coffee after a gourmet meal in a five-star restaurant. A man comes up and asks them how they like the coffee, and they enthusiastically reply, "We love it! It's so rich and flavorful."

When it's revealed that the gourmet coffee is in fact Folgers Crystals, the couple is astonished. "You must be kidding," they exclaim. "This is the best coffee we've ever tasted. Who would think instant coffee could be so good?"

The message Folgers was trying to send was that discriminating coffee drinkers enjoy their beverage. Yet there is much more to the ad than meets the eye. There's an underlying message here that you can put to good use in your dental practice.

No doubt, the coffee was okay. But it was the surroundings—and not the brew itself—that made the coffee taste so delicious. Would the couple have said the same thing if they were interviewed while drinking Folgers at a seedy diner? Probably not. It was the **experience** of the five-star restaurant that made the difference.

The newest incarnations of this type of ad are the ones for Pizza Hut's pasta dishes. The people and place have changed, but the message and moral is the same: positive experiences magically enhance the value of every product and service. People go to businesses (including dental offices) that provide outstanding experiences and gladly pay more for the privilege.

The Value Offering Ladder

In their excellent book, *The Experience Economy*, authors B. Joseph Pine and James H. Gilmore use the metaphor of a ladder to arrange the five types of value any business can offer.

Commodities are the first step on the value offering ladder. A commodity is extracted from nature and sold to the market. Coffee beans are a commodity. The value of the beans used to make a cup of coffee is about four cents. You can make money with commodities, but you'd better sell a lot of coffee beans. The commodity economy peaked in the United States about 1880.

Products are the second step on the value offering ladder. A product is made and sold to users. Procter & Gamble, for example, takes coffee beans, grinds them, and sells them under the Folgers label for about 15 cents a cup. The company can charge more because they add value to the commodity. They turn the raw coffee beans into a product people can use. The product economy peaked in the United States around 1950.

THE VALUE OFFERING LADDER

Services are the third step on the value offering ladder. A service is created and delivered to clients (or patients in a dental setting). Restaurants are a type of service business. They purchase ground coffee, brew it, and then sell it to customers. A fast-food restaurant may sell its coffee for $1 a cup. The fast food restaurant can charge more because it adds value to the product in the form of service. The service economy is peaking now.

Experiences are the fourth step on the value offering ladder. Experiences are staged and revealed to guests over time. Starbucks knows the value of staging experiences. Their typical customer comes in four times a week and spends an average of $4 per beverage. Starbucks charges more because they wrap an excellent experience around their high-quality beverages.

Major League Baseball has also recognized the value of experience. In every city where a fan-friendly, baseball-only field has been constructed—Baltimore, Cleveland, San Diego, San Francisco, and Miami, to name a few—attendance is up and the amount of money spent per person has soared. Oddly enough, the product itself (the team's win/loss record) actually went down in some cases, but the team rankings don't seem to matter. Why? The experience is what brings in the fans!

At this point, you may be thinking, "This is all quite interesting, but what does it have to do with me?" The answer is *everything*! Many of the dental offices I visit rise only to the service level. The problem is that all products and services begin to look the same after a while. It's this sameness that managed care encourages. After all, if one office is identical to another, then commodity-like fees are acceptable. The sad part is that as a result, patients won't demand a higher level of care *because they don't even know it exists!*

Now more than ever, the practice that differentiates itself stands to gain. You can differentiate yourself by going up a rung on the value offering ladder. Give your patients an experience. They will not only remain in your practice for life, but will recommend you to everyone they know.

Transformation is the fifth and next step on the value offering ladder. Transformations are as distinct from experiences as experiences are from services. **Transformations change people's lives.**

A growing number of people are asking for transformations these days. That's why plastic surgeons are doing so well while many physician groups are struggling. Plastic surgeons are in the transformation business. When dentists place implants and construct over-dentures that allow people to consume foods they haven't eaten in years, they're in the transformation business. And people will pay almost anything to have their lives transformed.

Moral Learned from the Value Offering Ladder:
Be in the Experience and Transformation Business!

Walt Disney: The Master Experience Creator

In the 1940s, Walt Disney took his two young daughters to an amusement park. In those days, amusement parks were slightly disreputable, dirty, and run by people who didn't seem to care. Walt asked himself, "How can this experience be improved?" His early answers were the beginning of the creation of Disneyland.

Walt knew the guest experience needs to be guided. And that experience certainly is guided for the tens of thousands of people who flock to the Disney Theme Parks every day. After you pass the ticket booths, you enter an area that is like the lobby of a movie theater. This area prepares you for the experience that is about to unfold. You walk down Main Street, and the excitement builds. You hear lively, upbeat music. You see Cinderella's castle off in the distance, which acts as a magnet to draw you up Main Street and into the park hub. Branching off from the hub are the four realms of the park. Just remember where Cinderella's castle is when you enter any realm, and you can use it as a beacon to find your way back to the hub. You are even guided in your choice of food. Ice cream wagons are often blue, signaling cool refreshments. Popcorn wagons are red, signaling warm treats.

In planning Disneyland, his first theme park, Walt always put his guests first. Walt told one of his park planners, "All I want you to think about is this. When people walk through or ride through or have access to anything that you design, I want them, when they leave, to have smiles on their faces." How's that for having a specific goal? When an attraction pleased him, Walt said, "I think they'll go for this," or "They're going to eat this up." His expressions of rejection were, "That's not good enough for them," or "They'll expect something better." Do you see how Walt was always thinking about "them?"

In addition, Walt didn't want other people's limited thinking to get in the way of the park exceeding the guests' expectations. To an engineer who pointed out the impossibility of one of his proposals, Walt replied, "You know better than to kill an idea without giving it a chance to live. We set our sights high. That's why we accomplish so many things. Now go back and try again." Those who worked closely with Walt learned to never say, "This can't be done." The correct response was, "Well, Walt, this might be difficult because...."

During his visits to Disneyland, Walt was always "plussing"—looking for ways to improve the experience of Disneyland and provide more ways to exceed the guests' expectations. He would study an area and tell his staff, "Let's get a better show for the customers: what can we do to give this place interest?" When a staff member questioned Walt's idea to spend $350,000 on an elaborate Christmas parade, Walt replied, "We can't be satisfied, even though we'll get the crowds at Christmastime. We've got to give 'em a little more. It'll be worth the investment. If they stop coming, it'll cost ten times that much to get 'em back.

In their wonderful book, *The Disney Way*, Bill Capodagli and Lynn Jackson describe the process the Walt Disney Company uses to exceed their guests' expectations. The first thing they do is create a *service theme*. A service theme is a simple statement which, when shared among all employees, becomes the driving force of service. At Disney theme parks today, this theme is an extension of Walt's original dream, which was "to use imagination to bring happiness to millions." Their service theme is, "We create happiness by providing the finest in entertainment for all people of all ages, everywhere." Notice that the service theme declares what the dream is (to create happiness), how the dream is accomplished (by providing the finest in entertainment), and for whom it applies (people of all ages, everywhere).

The Three Purposes of a Service Theme

What function do you think having a service theme could provide in your dental practice? You're office is hardly Disneyland, but without a doubt, your patients can always leave with a smile on their faces. Here are the three purposes fulfilled by a service theme.

1. A service theme emotionally communicates the purpose of the organization to everyone in the organization. In their book, *Built to Last,* Jim Collins and Jerry Porras say that a company's core purpose, unlike its strategies and goals, should be enduring. They write, "Whereas you might achieve a goal or complete a strategy, you cannot fulfill a purpose. It's like a guiding star on the horizon—forever pursued but never reached. Although the purpose itself does not change, it does inspire change. The very fact that purpose can never be fully

realized means that an organization can never stop stimulating change and progress."

2. A service theme is the benchmark for making all guest service and basic management decisions within the company. If an idea supports the service theme, it's usually adopted. If it doesn't support the theme, it's dropped.

3. A service theme creates the foundation for the public image of the company. All internal marketing, external marketing, and public relations must reinforce the service theme.

Service Standards and Delivery Systems

After you've decided on your service theme, you create your *service standards*. These are the measures of quality service that set the criteria for actions that are necessary to accomplish the service theme. At Disney theme parks, there are four service standards. In order of importance, they are safety, courtesy, show, and efficiency. In your dental office, a service standard could be answering the phone within three rings or stepping outside the office to greet people in the reception area.

Finally, *delivery systems* are created. Delivery systems deliver the service standards that accomplish the service theme. All businesses have three delivery systems: their people, their setting, and their processes.

1. **People.** Disney hires people with great attitudes and then trains them for skills. Disney says, "We don't put people in Disney. We put Disney in people."

*You can dream, create, design, and build
the most wonderful place in the world;
but it requires people to make the dream a reality.*

WALT DISNEY

2. **Setting.** In Disney terms, your setting is wherever your customers meet you. In dental practice, this would be your office. It also includes all contacts your patients and future patients have with any member of your team in a community setting, all telephone conversations, and your website. The importance of managing the effect of setting on the guest experience can be summed up in two words: **Everything speaks.** Walt Disney placed so much emphasis on setting that he changed the texture of the pavement at the threshold of each new "land" in Disneyland to signal a departure or entry because, "You can get information about a changing environment through the soles of your feet." How's that for paying attention to setting detail?

    Here are the components of setting at Disney theme parks:

    - architectural design
    - landscaping
    - lighting
    - color
    - signage
    - texture of floor surface
    - focal points
    - internal/external detail
    - music/ambient noise
    - smell
    - touch experiences
    - taste experiences

    Here's how Disney imagineer, John Hench, describes the attention to detail that's necessary: "Interestingly enough, for all its success, the Disney theme show is quite a fragile thing. It just takes one contradiction, one out-of-place stimulus to negate a particular moment's experience… take a host's costume away and put him in blue jeans and a tank top… replace that Gay Nineties theme with rock numbers… place a touch of artificial turf here… and a surly employee there… it really doesn't take much to upset it all. What's our success formula? It's attention to infinite detail, the little things, the little, minor, picky points that others don't want to take the time, money, or effort to do. As far as our Disney organization is concerned, it's the only way we've ever done it."

Do you pay as much attention to setting? I hope so. It's just as important. A good way to analyze your setting is to walk around the exterior and interior of your office as a new patient. Look, listen, smell, taste, and touch your setting as a new patient would. Have your team and your spouse do the same. Does everything in the setting support the image you want to project? If not, change it.

> *No chipped paint.*
> *All the horses jump.*
>
> **WALT DISNEY**
> (INSTRUCTIONS ABOUT THE DISNEYLAND CAROUSEL)

Disney calls the people who work in its theme parks "cast members" and their clothing is called "costumes." Every costume must send an "on-brand" message to the park attendees. Do your office costumes do the same?

There are no hard and fast rules when it comes to office clothing. For many dental offices, a great choice is to have everyone wear coordinated clothing, such as black or tan pants with comfortable matching shoes and button-down, collared shirts. Ann Taylor stores are an excellent place to buy this type of clothing.

Because of the surgical nature of my practice, I wear dress pants, dress shirt, tie, and long white lab coat for consultations and fresh, clean scrubs for surgeries. I wear scrubs only in the office. I never come to or leave the office in scrubs. The same is true with my team. They wear nice, coordinated clothing for consultation days and fresh, clean scrubs on surgical days.

3. **Process.** Processes are a series of policies, tasks, and procedures strung together to produce a result. These processes combine human (people) and physical (setting) resources in various combinations to produce different outcomes. All organizations can be thought of as a collection of processes. In the dental office, you have a process for answering the phone. You have a new patient experience process. You have a process for performing tooth-colored restorations. Each process involves different human and physical resources—and produces a specific result.

   It's vital that you identify the exact result you want and then construct the process to achieve that effect. If you just leave it to chance, the odds are very poor that the desired outcome will occur. Let's use a person's first phone call to the office as an example. If the result you want is for the person to schedule an exam appointment, you will create a process that achieves that result. If the result you want is that the person scheduling an exam appointment hangs up feeling that your office is different—that you really care about people and are a cut above—you will create an expanded telephone process that achieves that result.

Integration

Integration occurs when the cast, setting, and processes merge in pursuit of the service theme and standards. The result is an exceptionally high-quality guest experience.

Walt Disney's creation, Disneyland, opened on a hot July day in 1955. It was a huge success. Within seven weeks, a million visitors poured in. Attendance exceeded expectations by 50 percent and spending per person was 30 percent more than projected. Walt never seemed to tire of walking through Disneyland and watching his guests. "Look at them! Did you ever see so many happy people? So many people just enjoying themselves?" he would say.

One day at twilight, just before closing, a Disneyland employee was strolling through the park and saw a lone figure sitting on a bench. It was Walt Disney, savoring the sight of the paddleboat, *Mark Twain*, pulling around a bend in the river with a puff of white steam. His dream had come true. He used imagination to bring happiness to millions of people. In your own way, in your own community, you can do the same.

18 Memorable Experience Tips

Throughout the book, I've mentioned several ways you can stage memorable experiences for your patients. Here are 18 more that are on brand for most offices:

1. Send welcome packets to new patients. Don't include any financial forms/cancellation policies. Include your professionally done brochure and information on your services.

2. Provide rides to and from the office in a nice, clean vehicle for patients with transportation challenges.

3. Display a new patient welcome message on a sign or monitor.

4. Give comfort menus to all new patients, listing the special things you can provide them.

5. Burn scented candles in the office. Tommy Bahama makes candles with unusual scents. Order them at www.shop.bungalowbay.biz.

6. Take off your mask, eye protection, and gloves when you talk with patients.

7. Don't play commercial radio in the office. Play CDs or non-commercial radio.

8. Don't play cable or network TV in treatment rooms. Have the patients watch DVDs with goggles for long appointments.

9. Don't have TV or videos of any kind in the hygiene rooms. Talk to people and show them educational videos.

10. Offer soft pillows and blankets in the treatment rooms.

11. Have massaging dental chairs or massage pads on all your dental chairs.

12. Give gentle, reassuring touches on patients' shoulders or respectful hugs. This will convey caring more than a thousand words.
13. Provide warm, scented, moist towels for patient use after long visits.
14. Provide inexpensive folding umbrellas for patients to use and then keep on rainy days. The umbrellas can have your logo and contact information on them.
15. Make post-treatment calls to every surgery patient.
16. Pay for professionally done before and after photos of your especially nice implant cases.
17. Send warm, fuzzy, handwritten "just because" cards on a regular basis.
18. Mail or e-mail newsletters to your patients once a quarter. Include any continuing education any team member has completed and how the CE will benefit patients.

Conclusion

In the previous sections of this book, you learned how to take the first four steps to implant excellence: build a solid practice foundation, be a master marketer, make it easy for people to accept comprehensive implant dentistry, and keep your promises. In order for you to implement these steps into your practice, you're going to need to take action. Otherwise, all your good intentions and innovative ideas will fall flat. Take some more action now. Implant excellence awaits!

STEP 5

Take Action

WHEN CLIMBING A MOUNTAIN, a great way to begin is by picturing yourself on the peak. As you make your trek, you know the peak is at the end of the trail—yet you don't constantly look up at the mountain's apex. Instead, you keep your eyes on the trail directly in front of you and take one step at a time. Some of your steps involve trudging up a steep grade. Sometimes the trail will take you further away from the peak as you wind your way back and forth on switchbacks—but you're always moving up the side of the mountain. You encounter fallen trees and loose rock on the trail and sometimes the weather isn't the best. But you don't get discouraged. You don't quit. You just take one step at a time until you reach the peak and experience the joy of having transformed your vision into a reality.

Your journey to implant excellence will be a similar experience. There will be days when the climb is easy and fast—and there will also be days when you slide back a little. You will face challenges large and small. Some people and groups will aid your journey. Others may try to hold you back. But you don't get discouraged. You don't quit. You just take one step at a time until you achieve implant excellence.

Step five is all about taking action. It is the last and probably most important of all the steps, because the information you've learned in steps one through four is *completely useless* unless you take action to implement it. In Chapter 19, you will learn how to act like a leader by using six legendary leadership lessons. In Chapter 20, you will discover how to be flexible in your leadership styles. Chapter 21 will show you how to take action toward capturing ideas, setting goals, and creating plans. In Chapter 22, you will actively seek mastery.

You've kept your eyes on the trail to the peak of implant excellence so far. Take the next step now by flipping the page and discovering how to be a legendary leader.

CHAPTER 19

Be a Legendary Leader

LEADERSHIP AND MANAGEMENT ARE DIFFERENT. Leadership is doing the right things; management is doing things right. Both leadership and management could be classified as "the soft stuff," which involves people and relationships. The hard stuff in dentistry is actually performing the clinical procedures. The hard stuff is easier for most dentists.

In this chapter, I will present the six most important leadership lessons I've discovered:

1. Be a person others want to follow
2. Effectively communicate your dream
3. Team first, patients second
4. Create a culture of excellence
5. Make tough decisions quickly
6. Challenge unwritten rules

Leadership Lesson #1:
Be a person others want to follow.

Why does your team follow you? There are two possibilities.

1. **People follow because of your position.** Your position as the dentist and/or owner of the practice establishes you as the leader. The team follows you not because they *want* to, but because they *have* to. They need a job, so they do as you say in order to avoid the pain of losing their employment. They do "just-enough-to-get-by" work and will leave when a better position appears on the horizon. With positional leadership, you only have the potential to create an average practice—at best.

2. **People follow because of your character.** Their respect for and admiration of your inner qualities inspires them to follow. They want to be part of your team because it brings them pleasure. As a result, they do their best work. With character-based leadership, you have the potential to create a good or great practice.

I hope people are following you because of the second possibility. Because I believe character is such a vital component of implant excellence, I devoted the entire second chapter to it. In that chapter, you identified the five most important character traits you need to create and maintain the practice of your dreams. If you see your team is following you because of your position, I suggest you go back to Chapter 2, reread it, and begin to use your focus, actions, and surroundings to mold the temperament you need in order to become a character-based leader.

> *If you can become the leader*
> *you ought to be on the inside,*
> *you will become the leader*
> *you want to be on the outside.*
>
> JOHN MAXWELL

Leadership Lesson #2:
Effectively communicate your dream.

There are two parts to communicating your dream to other people. First, you must create a compelling dream practice; you did that in Chapter 1. The second step is to communicate that dream to others, because it's almost impossible to make your dream come true without the help of other people.

> *The very essence of leadership*
> *is that you have to have a vision.*
> *You can't blow an uncertain trumpet.*
>
> THEODORE HESBURGH

In 1961, President Kennedy didn't blow an uncertain trumpet when communicating his dream of America putting a man on the moon by the end of the decade. There were hundreds of problems (technical, political, and financial) that needed solving. Yet Kennedy didn't try to solve those problems in advance. He set the dream, gave it a definite timetable, communicated that dream to a team of knowledgeable and talented people, and let them try to achieve that dream together. The dream came to life when Neil Armstrong took his "giant leap for mankind" in 1969.

Like JFK, you need to sit down with your dental team and convincingly convey the following:

- exactly what your dream is
- why the dream is so important to you. Be congruent while using voice qualities and body language to add emotion to your words.
- what's in it for the team members. How will they benefit emotionally and financially? How will helping you achieve your dream move them closer to their dreams?
- what contribution you expect from them
- a plan for the achievement of the dream (see the next chapter)

After completing these steps and making sure your team has the clinical, people, and business skills they need, turn them loose to help you achieve the dream. They will respond in one of three ways. One, they will buy into the dream. You will see it in their eyes. Two, they will not be on board with you and will bring up all sorts of objections as to why the dream is a bad idea and/or can't be achieved. Three, they will be curious but unconvinced. They will have valid questions.

If any of your team members fall into the second category, they will actively or passively resist the changes necessary to make the dream come true. These people need to be given a career adjustment as soon as possible. It will be in their and your best interests. This isn't easy to do in many cases. I spoke with a dentist last year who said one of the most difficult decisions he ever made was to fire his best employee. She had been with him for over ten years. She was terrific at her front desk job, and the patients loved her. But she wouldn't buy into his dream, so he let her go. He went on to tell me it was one of the best decisions he ever made.

If any of your team members fall into category three, you need to get them actively involved in the achievement of the dream. Have them experience a few easy "wins." Keep the faith in your dream and in their ability to help you. Most of the time, they will come around. If not, they too will need to take their talents elsewhere.

An important part of the team buying into your dream is for you to understand their professional and personal goals first. As you learned in Chapter 12, you need to understand before you seek to be understood. Sit down with your team members individually and ask them two sets of questions.

1. **"What are your professional goals? How can I help you achieve them?"** I know a doctor with a hygienist who has a dream of being a national authority on the creation of training programs for hygiene efficiency. He's actively helping her move toward the goal even though its achievement will result in him losing one of his best team members.

2. **"What are your personal/family goals? How can I help you achieve them?"** Let your team know you care about them as people. Only then will they care about you and your quest for implant excellence. Often, you can use their personal goals as great reasons to buy into

your dream. For example, if an employee wants to be able to spend more time with her family, point out that your dream of a four-day workweek would certainly provide her with that extra free time.

Leaders touch a heart before they ask for a hand.
JOHN C. MAXWELL

Leadership Lesson #3:
Team first, patients second.

There are two groups of people who walk into your office each day: your team and your patients, in that order of importance. It's very easy to become totally preoccupied with serving your patients because there's a sense of urgency associated with them. ("We need to take great care of patients because they're here for only a short period of time, and they pay the bills.") I believe your team is more important, but there isn't that same sense of daily urgency associated with them. ("The team is here all the time, and they don't pay the bills.") But if you really think about it, without a great team your bills *wouldn't* get paid.

A great way to gauge if you are putting your team first is to examine what you do when a patient complains about a team member. Do you automatically think, "The patient is always right," then call the person to apologize for the team member's poor behavior? Southwest Airlines legendary CEO, Herb Kelleher, wouldn't do that. When asked if the customer is always right, Herb answered, "No, they are not! And I think that's one of the biggest betrayals of employees a boss can possibly commit. The customer is sometimes wrong. We don't carry those sorts of customers. We write them and say, 'Fly somebody else. Don't abuse our people.'"

Not only are Herb's attitude and action the right ones to take, how do you think his people react when hearing Herb went to bat for them? They respond with truckloads of loyalty that no paycheck will ever buy. In reality, when you put your team first and patients second, you will *increase* the level of service to your patients, not decrease it. When you treat you team with more care and concern, they will treat your patients with more care and concern. Everybody wins because you're putting first things first.

> *It's true that people can't be put in a neat box
> in a financial statement.
> You can't put a dollar figure
> on their net worth to the company.
> And you can't go to the bank and borrow against them.
> But people—not technology or fixed assets—
> are what determine the success
> or failure of any company.*
>
> ROY ROBERTS

Here's an excellent way to put your team first. Every Sunday evening ask this question: "This week, what are three creative ways I will let the individuals on my team and the team as a whole know they come first?"

Leadership Lesson #4: Create a culture of excellence.

In a 1995 *Forbes Magazine* article on the best companies to work for, it says, "There is growing concern that companies cannot live by numbers alone. The one thing that sets the top ranking companies in the survey apart is their robust cultures."

Your office culture is the invisible framework that supports and gives justification to the actions of your team. You can catch a glimpse of your culture by answering the following questions.

1. **How do you approach the workday?** Do you hate coming to work? Do you just tolerate your time in the office? Or do you thoroughly enjoy walking in the door almost every day?

2. **How does your team approach the workday?** Are members of the team routinely late for work? Do they seem to be just putting in their time? Or are they enjoying their days in the office?

3. **How does your team treat patients?** Does the team treat patients as objects to be fixed as quickly as possible so everyone can go home early? Does the team treat patients fairly well so they are satisfied with their visits? Or does the team provide your patients with a fantastic experience so they love coming to the office and can't wait to tell others how wonderful you are?

4. **How does the team treat each other?** Do they constantly gossip about each other and keep others at arm's length? Do they tolerate each other and treat each other well? Or do they love spending time together in and out of the office?

Your office culture provides your team's framework, but the individual pieces of that framework are values. Values are:
- deep-seated beliefs about the world and how it operates
- the emotional rules that govern your attitudes and behavior
- the guidelines you consider when making a decision

I hope you don't think all this talk of culture and values is just fluffy, sentimental stuff. It's not.

The greatest values are the farthest from being appreciated.
We easily come to doubt if they exist.
We soon forget them.
They are the highest reality.

HENRY DAVID THOREAU

Culture and values are two more examples of the "soft stuff" that are easy to forget. Here's a great way to make sure you and your team remember. Set aside 90 minutes with your team and create a description of the culture you want to create and a list of values supporting that culture. Now align your systems, policies, and practices with your values. Measure, reward, and recognize people who enhance the culture and exemplify the values. Periodically, examine your checkbook and calendar to see if the way you spend your money and time is consistent with your values.

In addition, consistently follow one of the most important rules of leadership: **Decide what's important, and then talk about it over and over.** Talk about your culture and values at your morning huddles, weekly meetings, and yearly retreats. Collect stories of people who have exemplified the values on your list—for example, a hygienist who provided outstanding perio care that healed a patient's mouth; a clinical assistant who went above and beyond to help with a patient's care; or an administrative person who brightened everyone's day with an unexpected and kind act. Tell these stories to your team, your patients, and your community.

> *The best leaders... almost without exception*
> *and at every level,*
> *are master users of stories and symbols.*
>
> TOM PETERS

Leadership Lesson #5:
Make tough decisions quickly.

Being an effective leader isn't always easy. It involves making some tough decisions affecting the lives of others. Unfortunately, many dentists avoid making the tough decisions and resolving issues. They sweep their troubles under the rug where the problems will be out of sight. And what do the problems do under there? They grow into bigger problems, and then mate with other problems to create a whole new family of little problems. Sadly, it's only when these problems become full grown and begin having serious negative effects that most dentists finally make the tough decision required to solve the issue in question.

*Again and again the impossible problem is solved
when we see that the problem is only
a tough decision waiting to be made.*

ROBERT SCHULLER

In the future, if you ever have avoided making a tough decision, call your team together and apologize to them. That's right! Don't get mad at them. It's *your* fault the 800-pound gorilla of a problem is rampaging around your office. Apologize to them for not taking action to solve the issue sooner. Here's how the conversation might go: "I called this meeting today to apologize to you for allowing our schedule to get so out of whack. We're all running around this place like refugees from the roller derby. We're not getting time for lunch or breaks. Beginning today, we're going to start controlling the schedule instead of it controlling us. In one month's time, we're going to be scheduled according to procedures, not time. I'll get you the training and give you complete control to make it happen. I really appreciate all you do for our office."

The tough decisions you make may involve a change in certain team members' responsibilities in the office. If you adopt the patient care coordinator position, someone in the front office may lose control of exclusively making financial arrangements. The tough decisions may involve an enhanced level of patient services you want to provide, or the entire office leaving town for five days to attend a continuing education program. So be ready for some resistance to your final resolutions.

The difficult decisions may involve pruning some prima donnas from your team. Prima donnas are all about me, me, me. Team players are all about we, we, we. If a team member doesn't buy into your decision, maybe he or she is a prima donna who needs a career adjustment. If you can't decide whether she should stay or go, here is a question that will make your decision easier: "If this person told me that she had found a new job elsewhere, would I be disappointed or relieved?" If your answer is "relieved," pull out the pink slip.

If you have a situation where two prima donnas are constantly bickering and their little feud is affecting patient care and is getting on the rest of the team's nerves, have a private meeting with the two. Tell them, "Laney and Doris, it's obvious you two aren't getting along. I like and respect both of you, but this can't continue. If you don't dramatically improve the situation in one week's time and keep it improved, we're going to meet again. At that meeting, I'm going to flip a coin. If it comes up heads, Laney will need to find a new job. If it comes up tails, Doris will move on. I'll leave you two alone now so you can talk. I hope you can work it out."

Listen to the whispers
and you won't have to hear the screams.
CHEROKEE SAYING

Leadership Lesson #6: Challenge unwritten rules.

We all have unwritten rules that direct certain aspects of our behavior. As an example, you may have a conventional belief about, "The more hours we work each week, the higher our gross will be." It sounds logical, but I know several dentists who have reduced their workweeks from five days to four and increased their gross and net!

Or how about the unwritten rule saying, "Busier is better?" Or, "The farther we're booked in advance, the better we'll do"? Both of these conventional beliefs are not necessarily true, and if you don't challenge them, they will place roadblocks on your path to the practice of your dreams.

The best way to challenge unwritten rules is to ask "What if?" about everything in your practice. For example:
- "What if we worked one less day per week and increased our gross?"
- "What if we didn't accept assignment of insurance?"
- "What if we only saw three patients a day?"
- "What if we stopped seeing children?"
- "What if we had a marketing plan where people called us on the phone and asked us to do their implant dentistry?"
- "What if we could do more dentistry with fewer people?"

> *In all affairs, it's a healthy thing now and then to hang a question mark on things you have long taken for granted.*
>
> BERTRAND RUSSELL

Conclusion

To say that your team members have dramatically different personalities is probably the understatement of the millennium. This is why it's necessary for you to Be Flexible in Your Leadership Styles. It will make you a better leader and make your life more interesting.

CHAPTER 20

Be Flexible in Leadership Styles

LEGENDARY DENTAL LEADERS have multiple personalities. Sometimes they're **visionaries** who move the team toward shared dreams. At other times, they act as **coaches** who connect the team members' desires with the practice's goals. In certain situations, they're **authorities** and execute a clear and decisive plan to move forward. Frequently, they're **delegators** who make it easy for people to do their jobs. And commonly, they **foster free will** so their team takes the initiative.

> *Stay committed to your decisions,*
> *but stay flexible in your approach.*
>
> TOM ROBBINS

I used to buy into the idea that the visionary style of leadership was always the best. I thought that was because most leadership books promote the visionary style. It may be the flashiest, but dental leadership isn't necessarily glamorous. Leadership is tough work. Flexibility is the key.

Flexibility in life is vital to our survival. Flexibility allows the coastal palm trees near my home to withstand hurricane-force winds. Flexibility enables chess masters to defend against any attack. And flexibility will allow you to effortlessly move among the leadership styles when the situation changes.

> *Nothing is more flexible than water,*
> *yet nothing can resist it.*
>
> LAO TZU

Leadership Style #1: Be an Authority

When you're recognized as an authority, things change. People interact with you differently. I know from first-hand experience. Being viewed as an authority in implant dentistry has opened doors, attracted opportunities and allowed me to accomplish things I never could have done without the authority label.

In this chapter, I'm going to discuss a couple basic principles of authority and then show you how to effectively use authority to your advantage.

Three Types of Authority

There are three types of authority. The first two are available to you as a dentist.

1. Charismatic Authority
2. Traditional Authority
3. Legal Authority

Charismatic authority is power legitimized on the basis of the leader's exceptional personal qualities or the demonstration of extraordinary accomplishment which inspire loyalty from the followers. Charismatic authority grows out of the personal charm or the strength on an individual personality. Apple Electronics' Steve Jobs and Southwest Airlines' Herb Kelleher are two business examples.

As long as the followers believe, the authority is intact. If the person behaves in ways that are not viewed as appropriate by the followers, the authority is diminished or completely lost. In recent years, many political and religious leaders have fallen from grace and lost their charismatic authority.

Traditional authority comes from tradition or custom. It is the authority of the eternal yesterday. With traditional authority, the rights of a powerful individual are accepted or not challenged by the subordinate. In many cases, inequalities are created and preserved by traditional authority. Clan leaders, kings and queens, heads of the family, patriarchal figures and royalty all have traditional authority.

Legal authority comes from the legal office the leader holds. Obedience is due to the office rather than the office holder. Once the person leaves the office, the authority is partially or totally lost.

Two Ways to Gain Charismatic Authority

You can gain charismatic authority in two ways with: 1) admired personal qualities and, 2) exceptional accomplishments. By all accounts, Steve Jobs was not exactly the nicest guy on the planet. But he did have two things going for him that helped him gain huge amounts of respect from the people at Apple:

1. He was an absolute fanatic at creating "insanely great products"—products that have literally changed the world. That admired personal quality attracted and kept thousands of the best people in the industry at Apple.

2. He achieved exceptional accomplishments—twice! As co-founder and CEO of Apple in the late 1970s, he built the company from nothing to be a computer industry leader in the early 1980s. After a dispute with the board of directors, he was kicked out of the company in 1985. When he came back in 1997, the company was close to bankruptcy. He led the way to numerous personal electronics breakthroughs such as the iPod, iPhone and iPad. In 2013, Apple's market value is more than the GDP of Poland!

From what you've read so far, I hope you see that Legendary Leaders have admirable personal qualities and have achieved exceptional results in their lives. As a result, they have abundant amounts of charismatic authority with their teams, their customers and their peers.

Gaining Charismatic Authority with Admired Personal Qualities

The first way you can gain charismatic authority is with admired personal qualities. This includes your basic character and how you present yourself. Let's discuss presentation now.

You have three charisma communication tools at your disposal: words, voice qualities and body language. Your **words** are what you *say*. They are actually your weakest communication tool. Still, you will want to have a decent vocabulary that allows you to deliver your message.

Your **voice qualities** are *how* you say it. It's your tonality, inflection, volume and pace. Voice qualities are your second most powerful charisma tool. Think about the most uncharismatic people you know. They typically don't have a lot of variety in their voice qualities. They talk in a monotone, at the same volume and the same speed (usually slow) all the time. They literally hypnotize others and put them to sleep. Now think of the charismatic people you know. Don't they have "jazzed up" voice qualities?

The best way to check your own voice qualities is to audiotape yourself when speaking with the team or patients. Then play it back and hear how you sound. The feedback is usually startling and instructive. Most people would benefit from adding variety to their speech patterns. Do that as you audiotape yourself again and listen to the improvement. In fact, stretch yourself and overdo the variety enhancement 20%. Then, in the real world, your voice qualities will be moved in a more effective direction quicker.

Your **body language** includes your facial expression, posture, gestures and clothing. Body language is your most powerful charisma tool. Legendary Leaders stand tall at all times, but especially in the face of adversity. Their followers receive the message loud and clear even though no words have been spoken.

At the height of her career, Marilyn Monroe was walking on a Hollywood street with a friend one day. She was wearing ordinary clothing, a hat and sunglasses. Her friend mentioned that nobody recognized Marilyn. Marilyn replied, "Watch this." She only changed the way she held her body and how she walked and everybody instantly knew who she was.

> *The world is like a mirror, you see?*
> *Smile and your friends smile back.*
>
> ZEN SAYING

You need to be Marilyn-like in your own way. Videotaping is the best way to do this. Your charisma is not set in stone. It can be learned. Joining a Toastmasters' Club is a terrific way to do it; or consider getting help from a friend or coach who understands the three communication methods.

The clothing you wear is also vitally important. I'm a real stickler on this one. The old saying that clothes make a man/woman is very true. The clothing you wear depends on:

Where you live: Well-dressed in Manhattan, New York is different than well-dressed in Manhattan, Kansas.

Your personal sense of style: I prefer a young business person style because it suits my personality. I have a very successful dentist friend in South Carolina who prefers the Charlie Sheen style with dramatic short sleeved shirts. He never wears a tie, but is always extremely well dressed.

An article entitled *Good Looks Mean Better Pay* on the CBS News website reported analysis done by the Federal Reserve Bank of St. Louis. The analysis showed that people who look good tend to make more money and get promoted more often than those with average looks. The researchers cited one study that found a "plainness penalty" of 9% in wages – meaning that people who appeared below average tended to earn nine percent less than those with average looks. They also found a "beauty premium" of five percent – meaning people who looked above average tended to earn five percent more than people who looked average.

The researchers couldn't be sure if the difference in wages was due to *external* favoritism by the people paying the wages or from *internal* factors such as the wage earner developing more confidence and learning more social skills.

A good way to think about style is to dress at least "a cut above" the other dentists in your area. To do this, I would recommend you getting some advice from a knowledgeable person in your area. Most salespeople in higher end clothing stores are more than willing to help you.

At First, Just Pretend

Adlai Stevenson said, "It's hard to lead a cavalry charge if you think you look funny on a horse." When I first read the quote, I didn't quite know what to make of it. I knew the statement was true, but I didn't quite see how it applied to leadership.

I think I have it figured out now. In order for dentists to be authorities and lead the charge to their dream practices, they must feel comfortable in their roles as legendary leaders. So the question becomes, "How do you begin to feel like a leader when you think you look funny in that role?"

The answer is deceptively simple: "At first, just pretend." That's right. Act like you know what you're doing. That will send signals to other people's brains telling them you're a strong leader. Just as important, it will send emotionally positive signals to your own brain just like the Smile and Look at the Ceiling Exercise you did in Chapter 10.

> *To pretend, I actually do the thing.*
> *I have therefore only pretended to pretend.*
> — JACQUES DERRIDA

Gaining Charismatic Authority with Exceptional Accomplishments

The first way to gain charismatic authority is with admired personal qualities. The second way is with exceptional accomplishments. Maybe you haven't built a wildly successful dental practice yet. Maybe you haven't even done an implant case. But getting the training to do place and restore implants is an exceptional accomplishment.

Many dentists don't make the effort to attend comprehensive, spaced-repetition implant training programs. Doing so makes a difference in their skills. It also makes a difference in their minds. They can feel it. Then their teams and patients feel it and naturally want to follow the dentists with high levels of clinical expertise. It's vicious cycle of success that enhances their charismatic authority.

Leverage your achievements by informing your community of the training your team and you receive. You can do this with press releases to the media and with newsletters to your patients.

Enhance Traditional Authority

Traditional authority comes from tradition or custom. Through the ages and in all cultures, healers of all types have held traditional authority. Contrary to popular opinion, health care professionals are still rated very highly—right behind firefighters and astronauts on most lists.

I hope your team members look up to you. They should. You worked long and hard to get where you are. You can enhance your traditional authority by belonging to dental organizations—being an officer is even better. Another way is to donate your time to community projects and/or holding a free dentistry day or local smile make-over.

Strictly Traditional vs. Legendary Leaders

In working with thousands of dentists through the years, I've discovered many of them are strictly traditional leaders. They believe leadership power is *solely* derived from their position in the practice. They think, "I'm the dentist. I went to college for eight years and invested $250,000 to earn my degree. I borrowed another $500,000 to start my practice. Nothing happens around here unless I'm in the office. I take work home with me. If I don't do enough clinical dentistry, nobody gets paid. I'm primarily responsible for my office's success. You should follow me because of my position in the practice." Almost all of the information presented in this paragraph is true. Even though the info is true, it's still not the basis for Legendary Leadership.

> *Being in power is like being a lady.*
> *If you have to tell people you are,*
> *you aren't.*
>
> MARGARET THATCHER

Legendary Leaders are different. They believe power is earned and willingly given to them by followers. Here are some other differences between strictly traditional and Legendary Leaders:

Strictly Traditional Leaders	Legendary Leaders
develop weak personal relationships	develop strong personal relationships
demand respect	earn respect
have tentative followers	have confident followers
have low levels of rapport	have high levels of rapport
focus on tasks first	focus on relationships first
speak first	listen first
expect to be served	serve others
have reluctant followers	have loyal followers
primarily use pain as a motivator	primarily use pleasure as a motivator

Leadership Style #2: Be a Delegator

Leadership styles can be thought of as clubs in a golf bag. As the player makes his way around the course, he chooses the best club for the current situation. When he is on the tee of a wide-open, longer hole, he chooses a driver. If the same type of hole has an extremely narrow fairway with potential trouble on both sides, he may choose the more accurate, but not as long-hitting, 3-wood. When he is 150 yards from the green and hitting into a slight breeze, a six iron may be her club of choice. Once on the green, he selects the putter.

If the golfer used the same club for every shot during the round, his effectiveness would be severely limited. The same is true with leadership. If you exclusively use one style, your practice will suffer.

Delegation Benefits

Delegation is the practice of turning over the responsibility for doing many of the key office activities to your people. Many dentists think of delegation as a task—an activity to be carried out and forgotten. In reality, **delegation is a process** making up an important part of successful leadership and management. To get work done with and through others, you must regularly give authority to them. Here are five benefits of doing so:

1. In the long-run, you save time and get more done.
2. When you choose the right person and give them the needed training, the job usually gets done better.
3. Your faith in people propels them to want to do everything better.
4. Your practice is more successful, and you're saner.
5. You deliver higher quality dentistry.

Of course, not all tasks or responsibilities should be delegated. You need to take care of the clinical and leadership responsibilities only you can/should perform.

> *When we seek to discover the best in others, we somehow bring out the best in ourselves.*
> WILLIAM ARTHUR WARD

Why Dentists Don't Delegate

In theory, delegation makes perfect sense. But some dentists have difficulty doing it. Their thinking process typically goes like this:

1. "Their ability to do the job won't meet my high standards."
2. "I can do it better and faster."
3. "So it's not worth my time and effort to delegate."

Maybe it's our basic personalities. We're perfectionists. We like seeing procedures done "right." But if we don't effectively delegate, problems pop up.

Lack of Delegation Problems

Here are five problems associated with lack of delegation:

Poor morale: A refusal to delegate can have a corrosive effect on the morale of the team. Good people want to contribute their talents to the practice in meaningful ways.

Burnout: Even the most talented, ambitious, and energetic dentists will run out of gas if they insist on tackling all major aspects of their practices' operations.

Misallocation of Personal Resources: Dentists who don't delegate run the risk of using too much of their time on routine tasks and not enough time on the important aspects of the practice's future such as strategic planning, long-range budgeting and marketing campaigns.

Damage to Practice Image: Dentists who don't empower their teams run the risk of inadvertently suggesting to patients that the team is not competent or trustworthy.

Damage to Practice Health: Micro-management often decreases your practice's ability to deliver high quality care to more people.

Micro-management Warning Signs

Dentists who don't delegate simultaneously stumble into the micro-management trap. Here are the micro-management warning signs to watch out for:

- Taking work home in the evening, working long hours or working on weekends
- Failing to give important tasks the amount of attention needed
- Excessive amounts of time spent going over/redoing work already completed by others
- Completing important tasks with little time to spare or a day or two late

- Spending inordinate amounts of time on relatively unimportant or routine jobs
- Frequently skipping vacations
- Having unhappy employees who tell you, "You need to slow down."
- Having unhappy family members who tell you, "You're a workaholic."

Keys to Effective Delegation

Effective delegation depends on your people being sufficiently talented and motivated to take on the responsibilities delegated to them. If the wrong people are hired, they require more basic training and supervision which invites more micro-management. Sound hiring practices and excellent training are major factors in laying the foundation for effective delegation. Once you've accomplished that, you can:

Establish a Positive Work Environment: Establish an environment where your team is not paralyzed by the fear of failure or look down on tasks they think are beneath them. Be sure to follow the suggestions in the three chapters of Key #4 to create a work environment that encourages responsibility.

Plan for Delegation: When you have a strong, clear vision of your practice's future, the role your team will play in that future and a plan for effectively moving to the future, you're far more likely to be successful at delegating than the dentist who doesn't do these things.

Review Responsibilities: Objectively examine which tasks you can delegate to others. Reserve for yourself those tasks which require the experience, skill, and training only you possess.

Select Appropriate People for New Responsibilities: Some members of the team are better suited to take on new responsibilities than others. When reviewing potential candidates, consider their motivation level, skill sets and emotional maturity.

Establish Policies: A detailed policies and procedures manual can help eliminate the uncertainties that slow people's performance of delegated activities.

Prepare for Bumps in the Road: Even the best-planned delegation efforts can go wrong, leading to short-term productivity losses. Risk is an inherent element of the delegation process, and some misjudgments may occur as people adjust to their new responsibilities. You need to reassure them that mistakes happen.

> *A company is stronger if it is bound by love rather than by fear.*
> HERB KELLEHER

Provide Training: Delegation of tasks and responsibilities is far more likely to be successful when your people have the knowledge necessary to fulfill their new duties. The fact that no one has the skills needed to complete a task doesn't mean you should avoid delegation. It may mean some training is needed.

Communicate Clearly: Be clear and concise when delegating. Right from the beginning, clarify what activities you're delegating and what you're reserving for yourself.

Be an Advisor: Make sure you keep lines of communication open at all times after delegating. Questions and uncertainties about their new responsibilities are natural. Make yourself available for questions. Be nonjudgmental and helpful.

The Power of Leverage

The best business people I know are masters at gaining leverage. They never think about working harder. They constantly contemplate how to work smarter - getting more "bang for your buck" in the same or less time. Delegation is one of your primary leverage tools. Like a lever helping you lift a huge rock, delegation can help you get more done in less time—and often done better.

You must make sure that what you're leveraging has a positive effect in the long-run. If it doesn't, you will create more negative results quicker. As an example, don't hire an associate if your current business model is not profitable enough to pay them adequately.

> *When you combine ignorance and leverage,*
> *you get some pretty interesting results.*
>
> WARREN BUFFETT

Put Your Big Rock in First

Michael Gerber wrote a fantastic book called *The E Myth* in 1986. It has been updated several times since then. The main message of the book is that small business owners typically don't spend enough time working ON their businesses because they spend too much time working IN their businesses. When you work ON the practice, you work on making the practice better. When you work IN the practice, you're serving your patients.

Working ON your practice is extremely IMPORTANT. When you do that, you shut your private office door, turn off the telephone and concentrate on your leadership and key management duties. Or you do the same and do training with your team.

The challenge with scheduling the IMPORTANT activities is that URGENT activities constantly crowd them out. URGENT activities such as seeing patient act on you causing you to be REACTIVE.

IMPORTANT activities require you to be PROACTIVE. You have the act on them. I recommend that you be PROACTIVE by spending two hours a week working ON the business. You must put these two hours into your schedule at the beginning of the week, and then commit to spending the time.

Here's a metaphor to drive the point home. If you had a bucket and wanted to put a big rock in it, you need to put the big rock in first. If you don't, gravel and sand will fill your bucket. Then you will make yourself feel better by saying, "I'll put my big rock in the bucket tomorrow/next week/next month/next year." Put your big rock in your bucket first!

Numerous studies show that companies having the highest quality and quantity of training also do the best financially. Join the group. Commit to spending two hours a week for 46 out of the next 52 weeks working ON your practice by PROACTIVELY doing IMPORTANT activities such as training, planning, improving your systems and marketing and strengthening your Core Values. When you do this, your practice will be transformed at the end of the year.

Leadership Style #3: Foster Free Will

Free will is the ability of people to make choices free from certain constraints. The existence of free will and its nature have been debated for centuries by philosophers. The debate is around the concept of determinism. Remember when you were young and set up an intricate pattern of dominoes in just the right way. When you pushed the first one over, all the other dominoes eventually fell. Some philosophers argue the domino effect is how human behavior is determined—that free will is impossible—an illusion.

Other philosophers argue that human behavior is directed to a certain degree by the domino effect, but that free will is possible and can partially or completely over-ride the domino effect. They say complete determinism is false and choices are possible.

"Choices" is the key word in the preceding sentence. Choice is at the heart of free will. I'm no philosopher, but my life experiences show me that free will is everywhere and choices are possible. I was very happy being a professor at the University of Miami. But a few years ago, I made the choice to head out on my own to start Implant Seminars and my private practices.

When I instruct the seminars, I see thousands of dentists in similar situations be exposed to the same material. Most of them make the choice to use the information to create better practices. Some don't.

I see my children make "good" and "bad" choices every week. I see them learn from the "bad" choices and not make them again.

Fostering Free Will at Zappos

In his excellent book, *Delivering Happiness,* Tony Hsieh says, "At Zappos, we think it's important for people and the company as a whole to be bold and daring (but not reckless). We want everyone to not be afraid to take risks and to not be afraid to make mistakes, because if people aren't making mistakes then that means they're not taking enough risks. We want people to develop and improve their decision-making skills. We encourage people to make mistakes as long as they learn from them."

Zappos' company policy is short and sweet: **Be real and use your best judgment.** And it's not just a policy typed on a piece of paper and filed in some cabinet in the company basement. It's a policy that governs all activities.

Most call centers are not pleasant places to work. Huge rooms are jammed with hundreds of people on phones using tightly worded scripts and rewarded by how many calls they can take per hour. Not at Zappos. When you take the Las Vegas headquarters tour, you will see hundreds of happy people working in cubicles decorated in very unique ways talking to loyal customers using no scripts. Zappos' call center people are not evaluated on the number of calls they take. They're evaluated on how happy the caller was at the end of the call.

The Zappos call center is open 24/7. One night at 1am, Tony and a few vendors were partying out of town. They all wanted a pepperoni pizza, but didn't know where to buy one. Tony suggested that a vendor phone Zappo's call center, not mention Tony's name and see if they could help. Within 90 seconds, the person gave him a list of three near-by pizza places that were still open!

Zappos also has 30 live-instruction courses almost anyone can choose to take on company time at no cost to improve their skills. They also have an extensive library of books their people can choose to take home to read and keep.

Life is the sum of all your choices.

ALBERT CAMUS

Choices

There are four factors needed to make excellent choices. As a leader, you must do your part to make sure the four factors are in place. The factors are:

1. **Knowledge.** It's impossible to make good choices unless people have the knowledge to support their decisions. Knowledge comes from experience and from training. Even though experiences tend to be the best teacher, people can gain decision-making references from both. So give yourself, your team and your family empowering references with a variety of experiences and with training. The larger the number and the greater the quality of the references, the greater is their potential to make great choices.

> *A man who carries a cat by the tail*
> *learns something he can learn in no other way.*
>
> MARK TWAIN

2. **Character.** Even if they have all the knowledge in the world, people of questionable character will make poor choices—often for dubious reasons. As a leader, you must place a high priority on hiring people of exemplary character.

3. **Freedom.** Even if your people have the knowledge and the character, they need to have the freedom to make clearly defined types of choices in clearly defined areas. This information must be communicated to them early and often. Failure to do so will lead choice paralysis… which is often the worst choice of all.

4. **Breathing Room.** Even if extensive knowledge is in people's heads; and they are of the highest character; and you've given them the freedom to make clearly defined choices; you will completely sabotage their free will choice-making abilities by punishing them for making honest mistakes – which they will sooner or later.

> *We need to teach the next generation of children*
> *from day one that they are responsible for their lives.*
> *Mankind's greatest gift, also its greatest curse,*
> *is that we have free choice.*
> *We can make our choices built from love or from fear.*
>
> ELISABETH KUBLER-ROSS

Mistakes

World War II had just ended. IBM's CEO, Tom Watson, limited his company's war-production profits to one-percent. He established an IBM widows and orphans survivor's fund. Returning IBM veterans could claim their former jobs. Gambling on a post war boom, Tom maintained IBM's employment levels by increasing inventories when there was little demand to justify the decision. With the end of the war, these inventories needed to be sold.

A million dollar government bid was on the table, but the sales rep failed to land the sale. The next day, the salesperson walked into Tom's office, sat down and placed his resignation on the desk. Tom asked, "What happened?"

The sales rep outlined each step of the deal, highlighting where mistakes were made and what could have been done differently. He ended with, "Thank you, Mr. Watson, for giving me a chance to explain. I know we needed this deal and what the sale meant to you."

The sales rep rose to leave. Tom looked him in the eye and handed the resignation back saying, "Why would I accept this when I've just invested one million dollars in your education?"

Experience is simply the name we give our mistakes.
OSCAR WILDE

Don't paralyze your office team by punishing them. Ask yourself three questions:

1. "Was it an honest mistake?"
2. "Is this the first time they've made the mistake?"
3. "Did they learn the lesson?"

If the answers are "Yes," be like Tom Watson—swallow your disappointment and support them as a valuable team member.

> *The greatest mistake you can make in life*
> *is fearing you will make one.*
> ELBERT HUBBARD

When You Make a Patient Mistake

When dealing with patients, your team and you are going to make mistakes. If this happens, take the following six steps.

1. **Listen.** The person you let down might need to get the disappointment off her chest. Don't make excuses. Don't interrupt. Don't even try to respond right away. Just listen.

2. **Own it.** When a team member makes a mistake, there should be no finger-pointing. Fans of Pixar's A Bug's Life know Hopper's first rule of leadership: Everything is your fault. Be sure the patient you've disappointed knows you understand the mistake belongs to you.

3. **Be humble.** Ask yourself, "Do you want to be right, or do you want to be effective?" You won't convince patients of your "rightness" if they feel they were wronged. You might be angry. You might be embarrassed. But you need to show them you are contrite and humble.

4. **Make amends.** Offer to fix the problem or patch things up. It's often the "little bit extra" you do that speaks volumes about your character. Doing an "above and beyond" gesture may even strengthen your relationship in the long run. I'm not suggesting you let people take advantage of the situation. There are unreasonable people out there. Don't give them what they want if it's completely unjustified and unreasonable.

5. **Be careful.** Just because you've made amends, don't think everything is back to normal. Be even more mindful of the disappointed patient and take great care to ensure your service exceeds their expectations. Until you get an unmistakably clear signal that all is well, stay in the penalty box.

6. **Learn from it.** True leaders learn from mistakes and use the experiences to grow. When you understand the consequences of your mistakes, then there's a much better chance you won't make it again.

Conclusion

As a leader, it's your responsibility to help people do the right things. This book is full of ideas on how you can recognize and do the right thing for your practice. In the next chapter, you will capture the ideas that you believe will work best in your office, and use them to set goals.

CHAPTER 21

Capture Ideas, Set Goals

YOUR JOURNEY TO IMPLANT EXCELLENCE BEGINS WITH A DREAM, which is why the first chapter of this book was about daring to dream. While reading it, you took five steps to create your dream practice. If you haven't done that yet, go back to Chapter 1 and record the steps in your journal or workbook.

Like Walt's Disneyland vision, your dream will magically produce several outcomes. It will:

- point you in the correct direction, acting as your global positioning device to signal you when you're off track
- give you the inspiration needed to make the journey even when the going gets tough
- put you on the path with other dreamers so that you can learn from and motivate each other
- bring you face to face with new opportunities that never would have appeared if you were just sitting on the bench of life hoping your circumstances would improve

In this chapter, you will discover how your dream will produce one more vitally important outcome. Your dream will be the magnet that attracts the ideas you need to safely and successfully complete the journey to implant excellence. Once these ideas are attracted to you, you must capture them and then use them to set goals. Let's discuss capturing ideas first.

Capture Ideas

I've studied dozens of creative and highly successful people. They all seem to say four things about ideas:

1. The ideas are out there, just floating in space, waiting.
2. They magically attract the ideas without any effort.
3. Their dreams, desires, and goals are what attract the ideas.
4. When the ideas appear, these people immediately capture the ideas by writing them down.

When I began writing this book, I didn't have all the ideas in my mind ahead of time. I just had a dream to write a book that would help you create implant excellence, and sure enough, the ideas effortlessly came to me as I worked on the project.

The same phenomenon is occurring in your life right now. You attracted the ideas in the book you're holding by your own dream of implant excellence. Dentists who don't have that dream don't have this book—or any ideas!

It's vitally important that the ideas you capture resonate with you. Don't select ones just because I think they're good or a columnist in your favorite practice management magazine promotes them. Your dream is unique, so it will require a unique set of ideas to achieve it. Only you will know what those ideas are.

> *A committee is a cul-de-sac down which ideas are lured and then quietly strangled.*
>
> BARNETT COCKS

Okay, enough with the philosophy of ideas. Let's get practical. Review the following bulleted list recapping ideas presented in this book and check with a pencil the ones you believe are most important to implement in your practice right now. Some of the ideas will be your responsibility to implement. Some of the ideas will be a team member's responsibility. You will further narrow your list and turn the ideas into goals in a few minutes.

Chapter 2: Character Counts

- ❏ Answer the question, "What are the five most important character traits I need to create and maintain my dream practice?" (page 21)
- ❏ Build those traits with focus, action, and surroundings (pages 21 to 24).

> *Money never starts the idea;*
> *it is the idea that starts the money.*
> — WILLIAM CAMERON

Chapter 3: The Dream Team

- ❏ Improve how you find people with great attitudes (pages 27 to 29).
- ❏ Improve how you select people with great attitudes (pages 29 to 31).
- ❏ Improve how you keep people with great attitudes (pages 31 to 37).
- ❏ Know the three myths about talents and weaknesses (pages 37 to 39).
- ❏ Discover talents in four ways (pages 39 to 40).
- ❏ Ask three questions to discover talents (page 41).
- ❏ Manage weaknesses effectively in four ways (pages 41 to 42).
- ❏ Realize that everybody has unique talents (pages 42 to 43).
- ❏ Use personality assessments to discover talents and weaknesses (page 43).

Chapter 4: Brand You

- ❏ Write your brand definition (pages 47 to 48).
- ❏ Collect stories that exemplify your brand (pages 48 to 49).

> *Ideas are the mightiest influence on earth. One great thought breathed into a man may regenerate him.*
>
> WILLIAM ELLERY CHANNING

Chapter 5: Be Your Own Marketing Expert

- ❏ Determine how many new patients a month you need to meet your goals (pages 59 to 60).
- ❏ Create a budget for your marketing (page 63).

Chapter 6: Intriguing Internal Marketing

- ❏ Use patient messaging software (page 68).
- ❏ Send a letter to all your denture patients informing them of your implant services (pages 69 to 70).
- ❏ Place a before and after photo album in your reception area (page 71).
- ❏ Hang professionally done photos of your best implant cases on the office walls (page 71).
- ❏ Show the ImplantVision animations and present a few of your implant cases explaining what you did, why you did it, and how patients benefit (page 71).
- ❏ Have your hygienist discuss non-hygiene topics at the beginning of the recare visit (page 71).
- ❏ Show 3D animations and narrated videos from ImplantVision's Patient-VU DVD to patients who need implants (pages 71 to 72).

- ❏ Identify problems that are caused by missing teeth and have a "would you like to explore the possibility of" conversation with the patients (pages 72 to 73).
- ❏ Calculate how much each loyal patient is worth to your practice (pages 73 to 75).
- ❏ Ask the loyalty question, "How can we treat people so they become loyal patients and are compelled to tell their friends and family how great we are?" (page 76).
- ❏ Make it easy for patients to refer family and friends (pages 76 to 77).
- ❏ Give referral gifts (page 77).
- ❏ Harness the power of the word "and" (page 77).

I can't understand why people are frightened of new ideas. I'm frightened of the old ones.
JOHN CAGE

Chapter 7: Extraordinary External Marketing

- ❏ Study the five components of an effective problem/solution advertisement, get some professional, unbiased advice, and start an external marketing campaign using traditional and/or nontraditional media (pages 80 to 85).

Chapter 8: Positive Public Relations

- ❏ Present direct-to-consumer seminars (pages 87 to 89).
- ❏ Stay in the public eye (page 89).
- ❏ Serve those who serve (page 89).
- ❏ Be polite to everyone (page 89).
- ❏ Use press releases (pages 89 to 90).
- ❏ Present lunch & learns to referring doctors (pages 90 to 91).
- ❏ Do a local smile makeover (pages 92 to 95).

> *The power of an idea can be measured by the degree of resistance it attracts.*
>
> DAVID YOHO

Chapter 9: Wow Websites

- ❏ Build a website that is attractive to the search engines (pages 98 to 101).
- ❏ Build a website that is attractive to the viewers (pages 101 to 105).

Chapter 10: Fantastic Phone Fundamentals

- ❏ Use the three tools of communication: words, voice qualities, and body language (pages 111 to 114).
- ❏ Develop your personal scripts for key office situations (page 115).
- ❏ Implement one or more of the 10 first phone call essentials (pages 115 to 117).
- ❏ Interact correctly with the four types of first-time callers (pages 118 to 120).
- ❏ Manage the time period between the first phone call and the first visit effectively (page 120).

*I am never so happy as when a new thought occurs to me
and a new horizon gradually discovers itself before my eyes.
When a fresh idea dawns upon me,
I feel lifted up, apart from the world of men,
into a strange atmosphere of spirit.
It is a new freedom.
I feel aloof from the world,
and for a moment
I am independent of all my surroundings.*

SOMERSET MAUGHAM

Chapter 11: Creative Case Conversation: Connection

- ❏ Change your mindset from "I'm the expert. Here are your problems. Here is what I think you should do to correct them," to "I'm a friend and consultant who's here to understand your unique problems, desires, and life situation. Given the information you've shared with me and my knowledge and experience, here are a couple ways we can solve your problems and gain your desires" (page 124).
- ❏ Create a patient care coordinator position in your office and revise your examination visit protocol to fit the position (pages 124 to 127).
- ❏ Be more likeable (page 129).
- ❏ Be more trustworthy (pages 129 to 130).
- ❏ Improve your levels of rapport (pages 130 to 131).
- ❏ Use the connection responder technique (pages 131 to 132).

Chapter 12: Creative Case Conversation: Understanding

- ❏ Have before-the-examination conversations with patients (pages 136 to 139).

- ❏ Have now-it's-their-turn-to-understand-you conversations with patients (pages 140 to 141).

> *There is one thing stronger*
> *than all the armies in the world,*
> *And that is an idea whose time has come.*
>
> VICTOR HUGO

Chapter 13: Creative Case Conversation: Education

- ❏ Improve your taking of records (page 144).
- ❏ Improve the most common handoffs in your practice (page 145).
- ❏ Improve your examination conversations (pages 146 to 147).
- ❏ Have after-the-examination conversations with patients on the comprehensive care path (pages 148 to 153).

Chapter 14: Creative Case Conversation: Solutions

- ❏ Have the solutions conversation for patients on the routine care path (pages 156 to 160).
- ❏ Have the solutions conversation for patients on the foundational care path (pages 161 to 162).
- ❏ Create your own dental care agreement (page 163).
- ❏ Have the solutions conversation for patients on the comprehensive care path (pages 164 to 178).
- ❏ Monitor the progress of your case-acceptance percentage (pages 178 to 179).

> *Many ideas grow better when transplanted*
> *into another mind than the one where it sprang up.*
>
> OLIVER WENDELL HOLMES

Chapter 15: Creative Case Conversation: Decision

- ❑ Respond appropriately when patients say, "Yes," "No," or "Maybe" at the end of the solutions conversation (pages 183 to 184).
- ❑ Have effective ongoing conversations with patients (page 184).
- ❑ Help patients do more quadrant dentistry (page 185).
- ❑ Frequently say, "Would you like to explore the possibility of…?" (pages 185 to 186).
- ❑ Create a toolbox full of patient stories to use at appropriate times (page 187).
- ❑ Create a collection of analogies to use at appropriate times (pages 187 to 188).

I could not sleep … when I got on the hunt for an idea, until I had caught it; and when I thought I had got it I was not satisfied until I had repeated it over and over again, until I had put it in language plain enough for any boy I knew to comprehend. This was a kind of passion with me, and it has stuck by me.

ABRAHAM LINCOLN

Chapter 16: Massage Money Magnificently

- ❑ Hold the seven empowering beliefs about patient financing (pages 192 to 194).
- ❑ Ask the nine questions you can use to evaluate financial partners and add a new partner if needed (pages 194 to 196).
- ❑ Use the 16 opportunities and methods you can discuss money (pages 197 to 199).
- ❑ Quote comprehensive fees with confidence (page 199).

Chapter 17: Provide Clinical Excellence

- ❑ Attend comprehensive surgical and restorative implant training programs with hands-on training (page 204).
- ❑ Create your implant philosophy and communicate it to your team (page 205).
- ❑ Obtain and use informed consent forms before all implant surgeries (page 206).
- ❑ Implement procedure-based scheduling in your practice (pages 206 to 210).

> *Getting a good idea should be like sitting down on a pin; it should make you jump up and do something.*
>
> E. L. SIMPSON

Chapter 18: Stage Memorable Experiences

- ❑ Create a service theme, service standards, and delivery systems to create memorable experiences for your patients (pages 217 to 222).
- ❑ Implement a few of the 18 memorable experience tips (pages 222 to 223).

Chapter 19: Be a Legendary Leader

- ❑ Consider whether you're a person others want to follow. If not, make some changes (page 228).
- ❑ Create and effectively communicate your dream to your dental team and family (pages 229 to 231).
- ❑ Take steps to put your team first and your patients second (pages 231 to 232).
- ❑ Create a motivating and nurturing culture (pages 232 to 234).
- ❑ Make tough decisions quickly (pages 234 to 236).
- ❑ Challenge your unwritten rules (pages 236).

Chapter 20: Be Flexible in Leadership Styles

- ❏ Be an authority when appropriate (page 240).
- ❏ Harness the power of charismatic and traditional authority (pages 240 to 241).
- ❏ Gain charismatic authority with admired personal qualities and exceptional accomplishments (pages 241 to 242).
- ❏ Use your three charisma tools (pages 242 to 244).
- ❏ At first, just pretend (page 244).
- ❏ Know the differences between strictly traditional leadership and Legendary Leadership (pages 245 to 246).
- ❏ Be a delegator when appropriate (page 246).
- ❏ Know the delegation benefits (page 247).
- ❏ Understand why you may avoid delegating (pages 247 to 248).
- ❏ Know how to spot lack of delegation problems (page 248).
- ❏ Pay attention to micro-management warning signs (pages 248 to 249).
- ❏ Use the keys to effective delegation (pages 249 to 250).
- ❏ Employ leverage to work smarter, not harder (page 250).
- ❏ Put the big rocks into your time bucket first (pages 251 to 252).
- ❏ Foster free will when appropriate (pages 252 to 253).
- ❏ Make excellent choices by paying attention to four factors (page 254).
- ❏ Learn to use mistakes to your advantage (pages 255 to 256).
- ❏ Take six steps if you make a patient mistake (pages 256 to 257).

Narrow Your Idea List

It's easy to get overwhelmed when selecting ideas. There are close to 100 ideas in this book alone. If you select too many, your brain will overload and you won't use any of them. Instead, choose the ideas you're committed to pursuing using the following guidelines.

1. Decide on a *maximum* of three ideas to implement right now.
2. Choose one action only for select members of your team. Be sure they buy into the value of the idea.
3. Select some easy ideas to implement first. This will help create the confidence and momentum you and your team members need to tackle the more difficult ones later.
4. Pick ideas from anywhere on the list, not just the ones at the beginning. As an example, you may need more clinical implant skills (a late item on the list) so that you have "the product on the shelf" when people call your office (an early item on the list).
5. Write each of the selected ideas on the top of a page in your journal or notebook.

Set Goals

In 1953, graduating seniors of Yale University were invited to participate in a research study. The graduates were interviewed and asked if they had a specific set of written goals and a plan for achieving those goals. Only 3 percent answered, "Yes." Twenty years later, the graduates were located and interviewed again. The 3 percent who had the written goals and plans had accumulated more wealth than all of the 97 percent who didn't. The goalsetters and planners were also more successful in other areas of their lives.

*The victory of success is half won when one gains the habit of setting goals and achieving them.
Even the most tedious chore will become endurable as you parade through each day convinced that every task, no matter how menial or boring, brings you closer to fulfilling your dreams.*

OG MANDINO

Use Your Ideas to Set Goals

Now it's time to use your ideas to set goals that are precise, measurable, timed, and planned.

Precise. Goals shouldn't be fuzzy. You should know precisely what actions are required. A goal of "Sit down and talk with patients before their exams" is fuzzy. A goal of "Have 10- to 20-minute before-the-examination conversations with all new patients in a private area using the suggestions in the *Implant Excellence* book" is precise. A goal of "Receive implant training" is fuzzy. A goal of "Register for and attend the next level course in Dr. Garg's Implant Seminars family of continuing education courses" is precise.

Measurable. The goals should have numbers attached to them so you know when they've been achieved. A goal of "Do a better job of presenting solutions to patients" isn't measurable. A goal of "Improving my case acceptance percentage 20 percent" is measurable. A goal of having a great website isn't measurable. A goal of having your website appear in the top three listings on the page when someone enters "implant dentistry Chicago" into a search engine is measurable.

Timed. Each goal should have a time limit for its achievement. A goal of "Improving my case acceptance percentage 20 percent" isn't timed. A goal of "Improving my case acceptance percentage 20 percent within six months" is precise, measurable, and timed. A goal of having a website link that appears in the top three listing of the page when someone enters "implant dentistry Chicago" into a search engine isn't timed. A goal of having a website link that by June 1st appears in the top three listing of the page when someone enters "implant dentistry Chicago" into a search engine is precise, measurable, and timed.

Planned. A goal that doesn't have a plan to achieve it is just a wish. Each plan should include the person who is responsible for the goal's achievement, the people who will assist the person, the resources required, and the action steps to the goal.

> *This is a story about four people named Everybody, Somebody, Anybody, and Nobody. There was an important job to be done and Everybody was sure that Somebody would do it. Anybody could have done it, but Nobody did it. Somebody got angry about that, because it was Everybody's job. Everybody thought Anybody could do it, but Nobody realized that Everybody wouldn't do it. It ended up that Everybody blamed Somebody when Nobody did what Anybody could have.*
>
> ANONYMOUS

You've already written your ideas at the top of your journal or notebook pages. Now, turn the ideas into precise, measurable, and timed goals with plans for their achievement on the rest of the pages. As soon as a member of your team or you achieves a goal, you can capture a new idea and turn it into a precise, measurable, timed, and planned goal.

> *By every part of our nature, we clasp things above us.*
> *One after another, not for the sake of remaining*
> *where we take hold,*
> *but that we may go higher.*
>
> HENRY WARD BEECHER

Conclusion

As you move toward implant excellence, several groups of people will benefit. Your patients will receive higher quality care. Your team and you will receive the emotional rewards of providing the best dental care and enjoy the financial rewards coming from a more successful practice. In addition, the quality of care in your area will increase as you show other dentists and their patients the benefits of implant excellence.

> *Not doing more than the average*
> *is what keeps the average down.*
>
> WILLIAMS WINANS

None of these benefits will be realized unless you become really good at what you do through the process of seeking mastery.

CHAPTER 22

Seek Mastery

GEORGE LEONARD, THE AUTHOR OF THE BOOK *Mastery: The Keys to Success and Long-Term Fulfillment*, defined mastery as, "The mysterious process during which what is at first difficult becomes progressively easier and more pleasurable through *instruction* and *practice*." Let's look at his definition one part at a time. Leonard says that mastery is "mysterious." As an instructor, I believe he's right. All of my students who are mastering implants are on different paths. Some students jump right in and do implants after the first two or three weekends *immediately*. Some wait until they have more information. Some students shift their practices to exclusively placing and restoring implants. Some dentists prefer to stay in the general dentist mode. Why does everyone do it differently? It's a mystery.

Leonard also says that mastery is a "process." Notice he doesn't say it's a goal or a destination. It's a journey. I've been placing implants, performing bone harvesting and bone grafting, and teaching others to do the same for over 20 years. I am happily seeking mastery.

Leonard goes on to say, "…what is at first difficult becomes easier and more pleasurable…" Placing your first few implants may be difficult. It might not be easy or particularly pleasurable. Big deal! The journey to mastery of a musical instrument is difficult, and it isn't always easy and pleasurable. That's why there are so few masters. The process weeds out the ones who aren't truly committed. This is why the vast majority of dentists don't place implants. Implants are more difficult than what they're doing right now, and it's not pleasurable for them at first. This is great! Their reluctance creates tremendous opportunities for you to separate yourself from the herd.

You're different. You've reached the last chapter in this book. I'm sure there were other activities you'd rather have been doing. After putting this book down at the end of this chapter, I'm sure you will take the next step to implant excellence. And then the next step. And slowly but surely, placing implants will become "easier and more pleasurable." And you will place more of them. Your patients and you will be the winners because you were willing to apply the dedication necessary for the journey to mastery.

Leonard completes his definition of mastery with "…through *instruction* and *practice*." Let's talk about each of these vitally important activities one at a time.

Instruction

In his book, Leonard says, "The search for good instruction starts with credentials and lineage. Who was your teacher's teacher?" I'm extremely grateful for the people who were my instructors in my dental school and in my residency. When I instruct students, I'm standing on the shoulders of my mentors and tainers. In many ways, it's they, not I, who are doing the teaching.

Leonard goes on to say, "To see the teacher clearly, look at the students." I'm proud of the 10,000 students I've instructed since 1990. The majority of them have taken the information in the program and used it to provide higher quality dental care to their patients. Many of them are my friends and colleagues to this day.

Here are two important messages when it comes to instruction:

1. **Instruction needs to be ongoing.** I love the continuum method of teaching. I want dentists to learn a chunk of information and then go home to the real world and do what they were taught. Of course, my students are always welcome to call me if they have any questions or challenges. And when a student finishes one continuum and needs additional instruction, there are higher levels of continuums available from *Implant Seminars*. This method of instruction sure beats a weekend class at the local Marriott.

2. **Instruction is best if it includes a hands-on component.** I believe in hands-on training that provides immediate feedback. That's why I've created many courses where dentists do procedures on cadavers or live patients under the watchful eyes of my faculty and me.

Practice, Practice, Practice

Remember that George Leonard defined mastery as, "The mysterious process during which what is at first difficult becomes progressively easier and more pleasurable through instruction and practice." All outstanding musicians and athletes know that mastery is not attained by doing 4,000 things a few times. It's attained by doing a few things 4,000 times.

> *What we do best or most perfectly*
> *is what we have most thoroughly learned*
> *by the longest practice;*
> *and at length it falls from us without our notice,*
> *as a leaf from a tree.*
>
> HENRY DAVID THOREAU

"He's Not a Walker"

You were on the master's journey as early in life as when you learned to walk. Your parents were probably the instructors who gave you ongoing and hands-on (or foots-on, if you must) training. You probably failed several times. You may have even resorted to continued crawling as a back-up plan. But your parents didn't give up on you. They didn't say, "I guess he's just not a walker." They—and you—persevered. You kept trying, until one day you walked while holding onto the sofa. Then you walked a few paces from one person's arms to another. Finally, you walked on your own to the delighted approval of your parents. In a few months, after a few bumps and bruises, you achieved walking mastery. Your journey was not a straight line; it was filled with fits and starts, of achievements and setbacks. It will be the same with your journey to implant excellence. As with all mastery, you will *not* gradually and continually improve your degree of mastery through time. That journey would look like this on a graph.

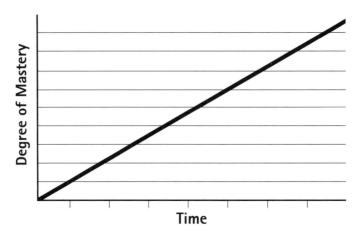

Instead, your journey will consist of brief spurts of progress that may be followed by slight dips, sometimes separated by periods of time where your mastery level plateaus and you feel you're not making any progress. The graph below illustrates what I mean.

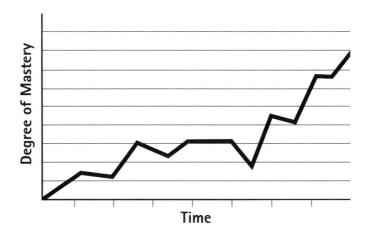

It's important to understand that the spurts, dips, and plateaus are completely normal parts of the journey to implant mastery. Now that you know what to expect, you'll be able to avoid three mastery-slaying decisions.

Mastery-Slaying Decision 1: *"I'm not going to start my journey to implant mastery because I'm satisfied with where my practice is now."*

I'm guessing this is the decision most dentists make. The problem with the decision can be summed up as follows: "You're successful today. Congratulations—you know what *used* to work."

The reason your practice is successful today is because you identified what worked yesterday and took action on that knowledge. The challenge is that the world of dentistry is changing. Not only are there new procedures that weren't around yesterday, but your patients have different expectations about what "good" dentistry is. Your own expectations probably have changed as well. So, if you want to be successful tomorrow, you need to know what's flourishing today—and I can guarantee you, it's not what worked yesterday. If you want to be successful in three years, you need to identify what will be booming in two years. From participating in the field of implant dentistry for the past 20 years, I can tell you that implant dentistry is thriving in many of the most successful practices around the world.

> *I will not allow yesterday's success*
> *to lull me into today's complacency;*
> *for this is the great foundation of failure.*
> OG MANDINO

Mastery Slaying Decision 2: *"I'm not going to start my journey to implant mastery because I'm afraid to."*

Very few dentists would admit to actually making this decision, even to themselves. More likely, they rationalize their decision not to seek mastery by saying, "I don't really want to do this." In reality, they're afraid of making a clinical mistake; afraid of what their colleagues or team might say; and/or afraid of spending the time and money it takes to seek mastery.

> *The greatest mistake you can make in life*
> *is to be continually fearing you will make one.*
> ELBERT HUBBARD

So what does it take to overcome the fear you may be experiencing? A little daring. Walt Disney explained his success this way: "I dream. I test my dreams against my beliefs. I *dare* to take risks, and I execute my vision to make those dreams come true."

Webster's Dictionary defines the word daring as "to have the courage necessary to take action." From my experience as a clinician and from my conversations with hundreds of dentists, I believe that the *dare* step—the courage to take action and do something different—is the part of the process that stops most dentists. They may have a dream. They may even believe they can achieve it. But they may not have the courage to act.

Why is this? I've thought about this fear a lot, and I believe it all comes down to one fact: **Many dentists will do more to avoid pain than they will to gain pleasure.** Many dentists want the pleasure of creating their dream practices, but they're not willing to accept the possibility of experiencing pain to achieve it. It's just human nature. It's easier just to keep rolling along the way they are now.

Think about it for a second. Where do you think pain can originate? Perhaps you fear it may come from your own dental team who may not want to change. They like the way things are now. Because it's familiar and comfortable to them, they will actively (or more probably passively) resist what you're trying to accomplish. It's hard to blame them. You've trained them to act this way. How many times have you come back from a seminar all fired up about implementing a change, then **you** didn't follow through and **you** let things fizzle out? After a while your team says to themselves (and often to each other), "Here doc goes again! Let's all *act* like we're interested, not do anything differently, and eventually things will die down (get back to comfortable) like usual."

> *Only one who devotes himself to a cause*
> *with his whole strength and soul can be a true master.*
> *For this reason, mastery demands all of a person.*
>
> ALBERT EINSTEIN

The second source of your fear could be pain caused by your intimate partner/spouse. Maybe he/she has rightfully come to expect a certain standard of living. Often times, the movement towards your dream practice requires an investment of time and money for clinical training, practice consulting, and/or equipment. Where's the extra money going to come from? Are you anticipating a reduction in staff salaries or lower rent from your landlord or better prices from your dental supply company? Not likely, right? Instead, the money is going to come from your net profit at first, because there's always lag time between the investment and the return.

Investment is the key word here. Your investment must create an enhanced return for you—an increase in net. Your investment must enable you to increase your fees and/or do more high-fee procedures. After the lag period, the investment will increase your net income and provide a higher standard of living for your family. You must be effective at explaining this investment/return cycle to your partner, or he/she won't be very happy when returns on their investment aren't instant.

The third source of potential pain could come from the insurance companies. They don't want you to seek implant excellence. They don't want you to be different and better. They want you to be a commodity so they can control the procedures you do and the fees you charge. They want you to be a cog in *their* wheel of success.

The last source of the pain you fear could be from your professional colleagues. They want to keep you as one of the group. It's more comfortable that way. If you change, the bar will be raised in your community. The rest of the dentists in your area will be forced to think about improving, and they don't want to do that.

Mastery Slaying Decision #3. *"I've hit a dip or a plateau on my mastery journey. This is too hard. It's not worth it."*

Take another look at Graphs 1 and 2 on page 278. Graph 1 is the way we wish the journey to mastery looked. Graph 2 is the way it actually does look.

Some dentists are dabblers. They approach each new opportunity with great enthusiasm, but become discouraged when reaching their first dip or plateau, and they quit. After quitting, they head out for a new opportunity and the cycle repeats itself. There are no quick fixes on the road to mastery. You must persist and learn to love the dips and plateaus.

> *I am always doing that which I cannot do,
> in order that I may learn how to do it.*
>
> PABLO PICASSO

British Prime Minister Winston Churchill knew all about persistence. He was invited to address the graduating class at Oxford University. When introduced, he walked to the podium and grabbed it with both hands. He paused for a moment and then looked at the audience, staring at the crowd for about 30 seconds. Finally, he announced, "Never, never, never give up!" Then another long pause, and with even greater emphasis, he repeated, "Never, never, never give up!" He stared at the audience for a few more seconds and then sat down.

This is undoubtedly the shortest major address in history. It is also one of the most profound. On the road to implant mastery, while sitting alone at night, a little voice in your head may whisper, "This is too hard. It's not worth it." Pay no attention to that little voice. Instead, tell yourself in a loud, emphatic voice, "Never, never, never give up!"

> *Twenty years from now you will be more disappointed
> By the things you don't do than the ones you did do.*
>
> MARK TWAIN

Be Smart

In addition to demonstrating your daring you will want to show off your smarts, because people who are just daring and not smart are dangerous to others and themselves. Motorcycle stuntman Evel Knievel was daring, but he wasn't always smart, which is why he broke hundreds of bones during his daredevil career. Here are five ways to be smart on your journey to mastery.

1. Start from Where You Are Right Now

Most dentists live on "Someday Isle." "Someday I'll take an implant course." "Someday I'll have the nerve to place an implant." You need to be different and start from exactly where you are right now—in your current location, with your current patients, and your current team. You will never attempt anything if you wait for all the obstacles to be removed from your path.

> *Whatever you can do, or dream you can do, begin it. Boldness has genius, power and magic in it.*
> GOETHE

2. Remember Who and What Is Really Important

On the journey to implant excellence, take great care of the people you love along the way. Don't get so wrapped up in your dream that you forget about who and what's truly important in your life. Seeking implant mastery is wonderful. Taking great care of the people you love is even more wonderful.

3. Take Care of Yourself

Seeking mastery requires the vitality that comes with eating right, exercising regularly, getting adequate sleep, and having some time for yourself. If you don't do these things and blow a tire on your journey to implant excellence, you could run off the road and get stuck in the ditch.

> *People who are too busy to take care of their health are like mechanics too busy to take care of their tools.*
> SPANISH PROVERB

4. Sharpen Your Axe

There's a famous story about two lumberjacks who were having a contest to see who could chop down the most trees in a day. The first lumberjack went into the woods and chopped down tree after tree, but never stopped to sharpen his axe. The second lumberjack chopped all day, but stopped every hour to sharpen his axe. Who cut down more trees at the end of the day? The second lumberjack, of course.

You, too, need to regularly sharpen your clinical and practice management skills by taking training programs that allow you to "cut down more trees" when you return to the office.

5. Help Others on Their Journeys

As you seek implant mastery, there are going to be others helping you. You need to return the favor by discovering what their dreams are, and then aiding them in achieving those dreams. If your implant excellence brings you greater financial rewards, share those rewards with your team.

> *All that is not given is lost.*
> RABINDRANATH TAGORE

Conclusion

As you make the journey to Implant Excellence, you will be a better dentist tomorrow than you were today. Your practice will be more successful tomorrow than it was today. You will be a better person tomorrow than you were today. Your patients will be healthier and happier tomorrow than they were today. And all of this will come about because you have made the decision to seek implant mastery. Have a safe, fulfilling and successful journey.

About the Author

DR. ARUN K. GARG earned engineering and dental degrees from the University of Florida and then completed his residency training at the University of Miami/Jackson Memorial Hospital. For nearly twenty years, he served as a full-time Professor of Surgery in the Division of Oral and Maxillofacial Surgery and as Director of Residency Training at the University of Miami School of Medicine. He was frequently recognized as "faculty member of the year" by his residents. Dr. Garg is the founder of Implant Seminars, the nation's largest provider of dental implant continuing education. He is considered the world's preeminent authority on bone biology, bone harvesting, and bone grafting for dental implant surgery. He has written and published seven books (*Practical Implant Dentistry: A Thorough Understanding; Bone Biology, Harvesting & Grafting for Dental Implants: Rationale and Clinical Applications; Dental and Craniofacial Applications of Platelet-Rich Plasma; Dental Implantology Dictionary; Implant Dentistry: A Practical Approach; Practical Soft Tissue Management for Natural Teeth and Dental Implants;* and *Implant Excellence*), which have been translated into multiple languages and distributed worldwide. Dr. Garg is the president of the International Dental Implant Association. He is a highly respected clinician and educator who has been a featured speaker at dozens of state, national and international dental association conventions and meetings, including the American Academy of Periodontology and the American College of Oral and Maxillofacial Surgeons. Dr. Garg has received numerous awards, including outstanding educator and an award for best article published by the *Implant Dentistry Journal*. In addition, Dr. Garg has developed and refined many surgical techniques and devices that simplify surgery while making it more predictable. He is a consultant and advisor to numerous companies. His private practices are located in Miami and Ft. Lauderdale, Florida.

Here is the sample Dental Care Agreement form mentioned in the book.

Dental Care Agreement

Name: _____   Date: _____

CARE COVERED BY THIS AGREEMENT
    Periodontal   _____
    Restorative   _____
    Replacement   _____
    Cosmetic   _____
    Other   _____
                      _____

INVESTMENT ESTIMATE
    Estimated Care Fee $ _____
    Estimated Insurance $ _____
    Estimated Balance $ _____

INVESTMENT OPTIONS
    1. 5% accounting courtesy $_____ courtesy = $_____ balance
    2. Visa, MasterCard, AmEx
    3. No-Interest Plan - ** months, $_____ per month
    4. Extended Pay Plan - ** months, $_____ per month

COMMENTS *(please initial each understanding)*

- I understand that changes in my treatment plan can occur. The actual fee may vary from the estimate above. _____

- I understand that my insurance coverage is estimated to be $_____. _____

- I understand that I, not my insurance company, am responsible for payment in full for all care. _____

_____
DATE   RESPONSIBLE PARTY

_____
DATE   DOCTOR OR REPRESENTATIVE

Index

A

action 4–5, 9, 15, 20, 21, 22, 23, 34, 37, 39, 44, 59, 76, 80, 81, 101, 104, 108, 112, 128, 130, 168, 173, 177, 182, 184, 187, 188, 192, 218, 223, 225-26, 228, 231, 232, 235, 261, 270, 271, 272, 279, 280
advertising (*see also* marketing) 54, 57, 73, 79-86, 99-100
    for team members 27-29
    sample ads 29
    problem/solution, five components 80-81
after-the-examination conversation 148, 156, 164, 182
    debrief 153-54
    sample for comprehensive care patients 148-53
agreement, dental care 157-59,161,162-63, 168,169,170-72 178, 266, 287
    samples 159, 163, 170-72, 287
amalgams (*see also* fillings) 140, 156, 160, 185
analogies 187, 267
Argo 25, 44
Ash,Mary Kay (see also Mary Kay Cosmetics) 59
attitude, of staff 25-35, 49, 188, 218
authority (*see also* leadership styles)
    Charismatic 241-42
    Traditional 245

B

before and after photos 71, 88, 90, 92, 94, 95, 101, 103, 117, 118, 121, 150, 151, 153, 157. 166, 168, 187, 223
before-the-examination conversation 136–40, 144, 155, 173, 176, 182, 265, 271
    additional distinctions 139-40
    elements 136-39
blog 97, 99
body language 188, 199, 229, 242, 264
bone grafting 72, 119, 275

brand(s)
   definition 45, 235
   message 64, 112, 220
   statement 48, 101
   stories 48, 49
branding 8, 44, 45-46, 50, 101,
   as a recruiting tool 49
budget
   patients' 70, 135, 141, 164
   marketing (see marketing, budget)
Buck, Pearl S. 211
Built to Last 217

C

Capodagli, Bill 217
care paths 156, 164, 198
case
   acceptance 54, 60, 68, 79, 86, 103, 108-9, 116, 120, 121, 124, 126, 128, 130, 137, 143-145, 153-54, 178, 179, 181-82, 192, 193, 266, 271
   four vital understandings 191
conversation
   after-the-examination (*see* after-the-examination conversation)
   before-the-examination (*see* before-the-examination conversation)
   creative case (*see* creative-case conversation)
   examination (*see* examination conversation)
   ongoing (*see* ongoing conversation)
   phone (*see* phone conversation)
   solutions (*see* solutions conversation)
   telephone (*see* phone conversation)
cast (*see also* team; staff; employees) 216, 220, 221
challenges 10, 142, 228
character 1, 8, 10, 17, 19-24, 86, 228, 242, 254, 256, 261
   three tools to build 21-24
   traits 21-25, 261
   sample description of 23-24
Churchill, Winston 111-112, 282

clinical
    assistant 34, 49, 88, 124, 186, 189, 207-209, 234
    excellence (*see* excellence, clinical)
    skills 8, 79, 101, 133
Coca-Cola 8
Columbo 177
Collins, Jim 217
commodity 47, 50, 102, 214-15, 281
communication, three tools 111-14
    body language 114
    voice qualities 113-14
    words 111-13
communication with patients (*see* internal marketing)
comprehensive
    care 61, 74, 126, 130, 147, 148, 156, 161, 164, 173, 174, 177, 181, 184, 188, 191, 193, 199, 266
    dentistry 19, 60,116, 142, 153,156,162,179,181,182, 183, 184, 185, 188, 199
    implant dentistry 10, 60, 128, 130, 149, 179, 200, 201, 204, 223
congruency of communication 114-115
continuing education (*see also* training) 13, 14, 24, 145, 223, 235, 271
conversation
    after-the-examination (*see* after-the-examination conversation)
    before-the-examination (*see* before-the-examination conversation)
    creative case (*see* creative-case conversation)
    examination (*see* examination conversation)
    ongoing (*see* ongoing conversation)
    phone (*see* phone conversation)
    solutions (*see* solutions conversation)
    telephone (*see* phone conversation)
creative case conversation 109, 123–33, 135-42, 143-154, 155-79, 181-88, 200, 265-67
    six stages overview 127-29
    stage 1: interest 128
    stage 2: connection 128–32
        liking 129
        trust 129-30
        rapport 130-32

stage 3: understanding 135-42
    sample understand you conversation 140-41
stage 4: education 143-54
    records 144
stage 5: solutions 155-79
stage 6: decision 181-88
    factors to "yes" decision 181-82
    responses to "Yes," "No," or "Maybe" 183-84
crown 149, 150, 152, 157, 166, 168, 175, 185, 186, 193, 208
culture, office (*see* office culture)

D

delegation (*see also* leadership styles)
    benefits of 247
    lack of 248
    versus micromanagement 248-49
delivery systems 218, 268
demographics 61, 64, 82
dental
    agreement (*see* agreement, dental care)
    practice 1, 4, 8, 28, 46, 48, 49, 51, 67, 69, 82, 85, 189, 193, 213, 217, 213, 219, 244
dentistry
    comprehensive (*see* comprehensive dentistry)
    comprehensive implant (*see* comprehensive implant dentistry)
    income from (*see* income from dentistry)
denture(s) 61, 68-70, 76, 79-80, 81, 82, 90, 131, 138, 150, 153, 166, 172, 184, 187, 192, 208, 215, 262
direct mail (*see also* media, nontraditional) 54, 80, 82, 85, 87
Disney (company) 8, 46, 216-20
Disney, Walt 216, 221, 259, 280
dream practice 9, 11–16, 21, 22, 23, 24, 25, 35-36, 51, 59, 60, 244, 259, 261, 280
    communicating to others 229-31
    creating description of 12–16
    sample description 13-14

E

Einstein, Albert 2
Emerson, Ralph Waldo 2
employees (*see also* cast; team; staff)
    selecting 26–31, 218, 229-31
    retaining 31–43, 231-34
examination conversation 146-47, 176, 182, 266
excellence, clinical 4, 203-212, 268
    keys to providing 204-210
experience(s), staging memorable 213-223
    tips for staging 222-23
expert
    dental 3, 16, 83,90, 92, 94, 124,130, 131,173, 265
    marketing 54, 57-65, 262
external marketing 54, 55, 63, 65, 79–86, 95, 111, 155, 197, 218, 263
extraction 161, 163, 206, 208

F

ffear
    as motivation 80, 101, 130, 279-81
    of dentistry 47, 108, 125, 147, 162
fee(s), dental 28, 50, 52, 73, 75, 131, 149, 150, 151, 154, 157, 159, 163, 166, 167, 168,
    170, 174, 177, 178, 190, 191, 194, 195, 198, 199, 206, 208, 215, 267, 281, 287
filling(s) (*see also* restorations) 113, 137, 138, 144, 145, 149, 150, 152, 153, 156, 157,
    165, 166, 168, 175, 176, 177, 184, 185, 186, 187, 208
financial
    arrangements (*see also* financing; payment plan) 125, 126, 148, 158, 169, 190, 235,
    coordinator 158, 189-190
    goals 59-60
financing (*see also* payment plan; financial arrangements) 141, 160, 267
    empowering beliefs about 192-94
    selecting the best partner 194-96
    ways to discuss 197-99
Ford, Henry 50
foundational care 148, 161–62, 164, 198, 266
Frederick, Carl 65

Free will (*see also* leadership styles)
    Choices 253-54
    Mistakes 255-57
        By your team 255
        With a patient 256-57

G

Gandhi, Mahatma 2, 24, 204
goals, setting 270-73
Graham, Gerald 33

H

handoffs 72-73, 145, 147, 158, 160, 169, 186, 184, 239
    hygienist to doctor, sample 186
    PCC to doctor, sample 145
    PCC to financial coordinator 158, 160, 169
    PCC to hygienist, sample 147
Harry Potter 1, 68
Hench, John 219
Henry, Patrick 111
high-end
    practice 16-17, 46, 47, 53,
    dental care 20, 193
hygienists 14, 28, 49, 59, 71, 72, 124, 125, 137, 140, 147-48, 184, 185-86, 189, 208-10, 230, 234, 262

I

implant
    case 16, 17, 36, 59, 60, 71, 85, 86, 90, 108, 120, 121, 223, 244, 262
    case acceptance 108-9, 121
    dentistry 3, 4, 10, 14, 24, 29, 36, 48, 53, 54, 58, 59, 60, 61, 62, 64, 67, 68, 71, 79, 81, 84, 85, 88, 90, 101, 103, 107, 108, 109, 116, 118, 128, 129, 130, 131, 135, 143, 156,

162, 179, 181, 189, 200, 201, 204, 212, 223, 236, 240, 271, 279
mistakes dentist make when helping people to receive 107-9
patient, ideal 61
philosophy 204, 205, 268
Implant Seminars Continuum 4
ImplantVision 71, 88, 90, 102, 162, 206, 262
income from dentistry 9–10, 36, 181, 190, 281
insurance (patient) 10, 28, 47, 50, 73, 118, 152, 157, 158, 159, 161, 163, 164, 168, 170, 171, 172, 176, 190, 211, 236, 281, 287
internal marketing 54, 55, 63, 67-78, 155, 218, 262
    ongoing communication with current patients 68-73
    in-office communication, six ways 71-73
    sample letter to denture patients 68-70
    work with current patients to attract new ones 73-77
Internet marketing (*see also* media, nontraditional, and website[s]) 54, 64, 84

J

Jackson, Lynn 217

K

Kelleher, Herb 231, 240
Kennedy, John F. 59
King, Martin Luther, Jr. 9

L

Las Vegas 46, 253
leadership 24, 38, 227-37
    lessons of (*see also* office culture, team, dental) 227-37
    styles
        Authority 240-46
        Delegator 246-51
        Fostering Free Will 252-57
Leonard, George 277
Lincoln, Abraham 2

loyalty
    cycle 74
    patient 73-78, 89, 123, 263
    employee 33, 77, 231
lunch & learn programs 90-91
    sample referral card 91

M

magazines (*see also* media, traditional) 82-83, 92, 94
Major League Baseball 215
management skills 3, 284
marketing 48, 50, 51-55, 57-65, 67-77, 79-86, 87-95, 100, 101, 109, 111, 127, 128, 182, 197, 236, 248, 262, 263
    budget 63, 82, 83, 84
    campaign 61, 63, 79, 80, 248, 263
    eight keys to success 58–64
    plan 54, 55, 57, 58, 59, 61, 64, 82, 87, 236
    external (*see* external marketing)
    internal (*see* internal marketing)
    tools 54
Mary Kay Cosmetics 59
mass media (*see* media, mass)
mastery 226, 273, 275-84
    -slaying decisions 279-84
    ways to be smart 282-84
Mastery: The Keys to Success and Long-Term Fulfillment 275-77
media
    traditional (*see also* newspapers, magazines, radio, television) 81, 82, 83-84, 263
    nontraditional (*see also* Internet, yellow pages, direct mail) 82, 84-86, 263
market size 80, 82
mass 82
Mother Teresa 2

N

Nike 46, 48
newspapers (*see also* media, traditional) 81-82, 83, 92, 99, 100
nontraditional media (*see* media, nontraditional)

O

office culture 48, 232-33
on brand 101, 105, 120, 136, 178, 197, 202, 220, 222
ongoing conversations 182, 184, 187, 188, 267
onlays 131, 150, 152, 157, 166, 168, 185-86
online advertising 97-105
online services, dentistry-specific 196

P

patient care coordinator 124-27, 140-41, 144-45, 147-153, 157-162, 164-169, 178, 209, 235, 265,
    Personality traits 126
    responsibilities 125-126
payment plan (see also financing; financial arrangements) 70, 195-96, 197-99
pay-per-click 100
PCC (*see* patient care coordinator)
phone
    conversations with patients 54, 64, 108, 109, 111-121, 128, 131, 136, 182, 196, 197-99, 218, 219, 221, 264
    first call essentials 115-17
    four types of first-time callers 118-20
    sample call with price shopper 119
    scripts (see scripts, for telephone calls)
photographing patients 71, 88, 90, 94, 140, 206,
photos, before and after (*see* before and after photos)
Pine, B. Joseph 214
Porras, Jerry 217
PowerPoint 88, 90, 175

practice
    foundation 4, 5, 7–8, 17, 105, 107, 200, 201, 223
    cornerstones of a solid practice foundation 7-8
    management 1, 3–4, 24, 58, 79, 126, 193, 188, 284
    management software 68, 178-79, 196
    vision 9, 10, 11, 15, 31, 225, 229, 249, 259
press release 89-90, 245
privacy policy 104
problem/solution advertising message (*see* advertising, problem/solution message)
psychographics 61, 64
public relations 48, 54-55, 63, 64, 65, 86, 87-95, 101, 107, 111, 155, 201, 218, 263
    strategies (*see also* seminars, direct to consumer, press release, lunch & learn, smile makeover) 87-95

Q

quadrant dentistry 185-86, 267

R

radio (*see also* media, traditional) 49, 54, 80, 83, 92, 93, 95, 99, 100, 222
radiographs 125, 144
rapport 62, 99, 129, 130-32, 246, 265
recare 36, 68-71, 75, 104, 184, 185, 199, 209-10, 262
return on investment (*see* ROI)
referrals, of patients 46, 54, 76, 77, 90, 101,138, 205, 263
    gifts 75, 77
    of new patients from current ones 73-74
restorations (*see also* fillings) 94, 112, 113, 125, 131, 138, 140, 141, 147, 150, 151, 157, 158, 159, 166, 167, 168, 170, 171, 172, 176, 177, 184, 185, 186, 188, 205, 208, 221
Roberts, Julia 103, 129,
Robbins, Tony 2
ROI (return on investment) 81, 86
root canal 137, 140, 144-46, 149, 161, 163, 166, 175, 183-84
routine care 147, 148, 156-60, 198, 266
Rowling, J.K. 68

S

scheduling, patient 9, 14, 63, 64, 68, 76, 87, 88, 92, 94, 104, 112, 117, 118, 120, 153, 154, 158, 160, 169, 178, 183, 193, 199, 204, 206-10, 221, 268
    checklist for procedure-based 207-10
    sample of procedure-based schedule 209
Schweitzer, Albert 2
scripts, for telephone calls 64, 115-18, 197, 253
search engines 84-85, 95, 97-101, 238, 244, 264, 272
    eight tips to build website attractive to 98-100
seminars
    direct-to-consumer 87-89, 237
    Implant 2, 4, 9, 63, 204, 252, 271, 276
service
    delivery systems 217–22, 268
    integration 217-18
    standards 218, 268
    theme, purposes 217-18, 268
smile
    makeover 92-95, 263
solutions conversation 140, 148, 156, 150–73, 174, 176, 177, 178, 181, 182, 183, 266, 267
    points for comprehensive care 174-78
    points for foundational care 162
    points for routine care 160
    sample for comprehensive care path patients 164-172
    sample for foundational care path patients 161-63
    sample for routine care path patients 156-58
    steps for comprehensive care path patients 173-74
Southwest Airlines 48, 231, 240
    company values 231
sponsored links 99-100
staff (*see also* employees; cast; team) 10, 13, 20, 22, 32, 35, 37, 69, 70, 112, 113
Starbucks 46, 215
stories, patient, four parts 187

T

Tap Scan Reports 83
team (*see also* staff; cast; employee)
    dental 1, 4, 5, 8, 10, 12, 13, 14, 19, 20, 22, 23, 24, 25-44, 41, 45, 46, 49, 52, 54, 65, 68, 69, 70, 71–72, 78, 82, 83, 84, 85, 94, 96, 97, 101, 102, 103, 106, 107, 108–15, 119–27, 129–30, 133, 134, 139, 144–45, 168–73, 179–80, 182, 183, 185, 191–94, 199, 200, 204, 205, 213–14, 217, 221–32, 235, 241–43, 245, 246, 253–54, 256, 257
    finding team members 27-29
    retaining team members 31-37
    selecting team members 29-31
telephone conversations (*see* phone conversations)
television (TV) (*see also* media, traditional) 54, 62, 80, 82, 83-84, 92, 95, 99, 100, 177, 222
testimonials 71, 99, 101, 104
The DisneyWay 217
The Experience Economy 214
The Secret 5
The Wizard of Oz 1, 11–12, 15
Tracy, Brian 2
traditional media (*see* media, traditional)
training (*see also* continuing education)
    dental 16, 52, 89-90, 94, 125, 131, 198, 204, 244-45, 268
    dental team 35, 40, 42, 109, 115, 230, 235, 247, 249, 250, 251, 253
    restorative implant 57, 204, 268
treatment
    conference 108, 125, 126, 140, 173, 189, 190
    plan(s) 60, 84, 108, 116, 125, 135, 147, 148, 152, 174, 181, 193
        good, better, best 170-72, 174, 177, 199

U

University of Miami 3, 57, 252

V

value offering ladder 214-15
values 50, 61, 233-34, 251
Values and Lifestyle Survey 61
    four population groups 61-63
        achievers 62
        belongers 61
        emulators 62
        socially conscious 62-63
veneers 151-53, 168, 174, 175, 177, 186
Versace 8
vision, practice (*see* practice vision)
voice qualities 111, 113-14, 115, 199, 229, 242, 264

W

Web marketing company 100
website(s) (*see also* media, nontraditional, and Internet marketing) 54, 65, 81, 82,
    84-85, 95, 97–105, 111, 117, 119, 120, 121, 155, 197, 219, 243, 264
    10 tips to build a viewer-attracting implant 101-205
whitening 89, 151, 152, 167–72, 174
Woods, Tiger 201-202
World Trade Center 20

Y

yellow pages (*see also* media, nontraditional) 80, 82, 85, 97

Z

Ziglar, Zig 2
Zappos 252-53

Notes

Notes